# *But You Don't Look Sick!*

## *Fibromyalgia Facts and True Stories*

**Bette Brown**

**Note:** *All medical information included in this book is based on a personal experience. For questions or concerns regarding health or diagnoses, please consult a doctor or a medical professional.*

# *Dedication*

I dedicate this book to my sister, Mary and daughter, Genna. Both are warriors, fighting their own personal battle with an invisible illness.

# *Acknowledgements*

I would like to thank my dear friend, Ann Holliday, for her unequivocal support and friendship throughout for which my mere expression of thanks does not satisfy. Her critique and advice have been invaluable. My gratitude further extends to my Copywriter Jesse Mills, Thank you both.

# Contents

# A Brief Introduction

I assume that if you have purchased this small book you are seeking information on the painful disorder Fibromyalgia or Fibromyalgia Syndrome (FMS).

The aim of this book is not for a self-diagnosis, nor is it to direct you into a prospective self-treatment. If you suspect you may have FMS yourself seek testing, diagnosis and treatment from a qualified medical professional; with your General Practitioner (GP) being the best first step.

This book may be a go-to guide if you are an existing sufferer and may offer you a few tips to help manage your FMS better, or it may give you food for thought around the wellbeing of a loved one. My hope is the reader will gain a better understanding of this debilitating illness.

FMS is an unforgiving and incurable illness which causes varying degrees of inexplicable pain throughout many areas of the body. It can affect adults, the elderly and even children, but it's most likely to affect females, aged between thirty and fifty years old.

They diagnose one in twenty people in the UK with FMS. In terms of a numerical value, this translates to being around 1.5 and 2 million suffers of FMS in the United Kingdom alone.

In the United States of America, research suggests that FMS is just as prevalent, with 10 million sufferers, and to put the size of this disorder into a global perspective, somewhere between three and five percent of the world's population receives a diagnosis of FMS.

Many people receive an FMS diagnosis daily and most do not understand how this illness will impact their lives. I wrote this book to share my research and knowledge on the subject.

I have written this work in two distinct parts. Part one offers the reader information, advice and tips on various topics including childhood Juvenile Fibromyalgia Syndrome, JFS.

Part two comprises of true stories from people diagnosed with FMS and how they cope with everyday living. I found this part challenging and upsetting to write. We never know what people endure or the reason they develop this gruelling illness.

It is my hope you find something of value which may aid you or educate your family on this debilitating disorder.

# Chapter 1
# What is Fibromyalgia?

The word "Fibro" relates to the fibrous tissues such as tendons and ligaments found in our joints, and "myalgia" refers to pain, so the term Fibromyalgia means pain in the joints and muscles.

It is an unrelenting disorder which affects every part of your life. This illness burrows deep into your body, poking its head up wherever and whenever it pleases and has its own set of ever-changing rules. It may or may not respond to mainstream medications and it subjects you too many coexisting illnesses.

We know FMS as a syndrome because it amalgamates several symptoms. Pain and fatigue sufferers often experience unrefreshing sleep, insomnia and copious bouts of fatigue.

The debilitating pain of FMS may come and go at random with no pattern or routine and does not discriminate against which part of the body it attacks. The pain can vary in severity from mild to severe. It may attack any area, but it's most noted for affecting mobile areas such as the waist, back, shoulders, neck, chest, and joints such as the knees and elbows.

Perhaps the second biggest physical symptom of FMS are the feelings of Chronic Fatigue Syndrome (CFS) This can often range in severity from feeling a little weary and tired to a full-blown state of exhaustion. It can come and go at random. Sufferers often describe how they feel devoid of energy, almost as if someone had just "flicked a switch" or "pulled the plug" on them. This level of fatigue affects their daily life and cannot improve by catching up on their rest and sleep. They may still feel fatigued after sleeping solidly for twelve hours or more.

During my research I discovered that people who suffer with mild-to-moderate experiences of FMS can live a normal life when given the correct support and treatment. Those who experience high extreme pain may have learned strategies to live life with the disorder and may rely on natural remedies and prescription medications to obtain a decent quality of life.

## What Causes Fibromyalgia?

The true cause of the pain that typifies FMS is unknown although it's thought that a chemical imbalance in the brain, a genetic fault, or a trauma is the culprit. People with this illness often have low levels of the hormones **Serotine** and **Dopamine** in their brain.

Low levels of these hormones may trigger FMS as they regulate your moods, stress levels, appetite, behaviour and play a role on how you manage pain messages. But there is no real sign of why one group of people should get the disorder and others do not. What we know is people with this debilitating disorder have an increased sensitivity to pain, or a "glitch" in the way the brain processes pain.

Medical professionals can't agree on the root cause of the illness They have various theories, but there is no concrete evidence to pinpoint a specific cause. Some doctors believe that various life events may be so traumatic that they change how our brains translate pain.

People have opposing ideas on what they may consider a traumatic occurrence. We each differ in our thoughts and opinions, while a percentage of people recover from stress it may take other individuals, years to accept and move on from a past trauma.

## How do we get Fibromyalgia?

It is unclear why a percentage of people contract FMS, but it involves many considerations, with mental, physical and emotional stress being one key to the onset of this illness. If you are an FMS sufferer, it is likely you have experienced a traumatic life event, although a small percentage of people develop this illness with no known cause or reason.

The NHS UK suggest any of the following events may trigger our response to pain and may onset FMS.
*A stressful birth
*An abusive relationship
*The sudden death of a loved one
*A viral infection
*An accident
*A divorce
*A serious injury
*PTSS
*Surgery
*Genetics
If you assume you have FMS it's important you receive a diagnosis, medication and a management plan.

## A Diagnosis

Be prepared for a long drawn out wait as many doctors are unsympathetic. They assume depression is the root cause of ill health, or even refuse to accept that FMS exists even though the government has now recognised the illness as a chronic pain medical disorder.

FMS is not a new medical condition but for most of the last century it was problematic to diagnose with standard laboratory tests or X-rays, as many of the symptoms of the illness are present in other conditions with chronic fatigue syndrome (CFS) being a good example.

An early 1970s study into FMS came to the forefront when a pair of Canadian doctors developed a way of diagnosing FMS and by 1990, an international committee created and published the requirements for a diagnosis. This very much depends on your how severe the pain is and how long it has been present.

A rheumatologist or GP may diagnose you with the disorder if you have experienced inexplicable pain for over three months, in at least 11 out of 18 tender points. The recognised tender points are, at the back of the neck, the elbows, the knees, the front of the neck, the hips, the lower and upper parts of the back, the shoulders, buttocks and the chest on both sides of the body. A GP may manipulate these areas with a reasonable force to diagnose you.

It can take years for a diagnosis and to receive the correct treatment. The first initial step is to visit your doctor. Tell him/her all your symptoms. It is important you describe each problem you are experiencing in depth and stress that your pain is widespread and not localised.

Your doctor should carry out a series of tests to check any underlying problems. These tests are to dismiss similar illnesses such as, rheumatic or neurological disorders which may mimic FMS. It's normal to investigate these conditions first before looking into why you experience widespread pain. If the results return negative, then your GP may suggest a referral to a rheumatologist for final confirmation of the disorder.

Often a genetic cause is dominant in a few patients with FMS and your doctor may want information on other members of your immediate family who experience similar symptoms. They may even ask if you suffer from any mental health issues.

In the next chapter, we will look at some coexisting illness that accompany FMS, which may add further misery to a sufferer's daily life.

# Chapter 2
# **Coexisting Disorders**

FMS may be difficult to diagnose and is often mistaken for other comorbid disorders.

It is impossible to include every condition known to coexist with the disorder, so I have listed the most common illnesses most sufferers experience. I am sure that most people with FMS have experienced several, if not more, of these coexisting illnesses.

FMS is a harsh illness. It not only plagues the sufferer with extreme pain but throws many coexisting disorders into the mix, making the illness harder to endure and often rendering the sufferer incapable of functioning.

**\*Sleep Disturbances:**
Insomnia and sleep disturbances are a key clinical part of FMS, Symptoms may range from restlessness, tossing and turning, to full blown insomnia where the patient may lay awake for hours. A lack of restoring sleep renders a sufferer to experience even more pain.

**\*Chronic Fatigue Syndrome:**
This is the extreme tiredness we discussed earlier. It may occur with or without widespread pain. It is a debilitating illness on its own without the added extra of FMS. As well as the debilitating fatigue and unrefreshing sleep, there is the worsening of symptoms after exertion.

## Costochondritis:

*This unpleasant disorder is inflammation of the cartilage in the rib cage, it normally affects the cartilage where the upper ribs attach to the breastbone.

*Pain caused by costochondritis can range from mild to severe. Mild cases may cause your chest to feel tender. Severe cases may cause shooting pains down your arms or uncomfortable chest pains. The condition often goes away within a few weeks, but some cases may require treatment.

*People with costochondritis often experience pain in the upper and middle rib area on either side of the breastbone. The pain may radiate to the back or the abdomen. It may also get worse if you move, stretch or breathe deeply. This disorder can mimic a heart attack.

*All chest pain should be discussed with a medical professional.

## *Restless Leg Syndrome:

FMS patients have described this limb movement disorder as a crawling sensation and pain in both the calves and feet. It causes the sufferer an overwhelming urge to move their legs. RLS worsens at night and often it's impossible to find a comfortable resting place. It eases while you are awake. There needs more research to find the underlying cause of this symptom.

## *Irritable Bowel Syndrome:

IBS, acid reflux, diarrhoea and/or constipation, are common coexisting illnesses which causes nausea, gas, bloating and abdominal extension.

*It is important to seek medical help if you experience any symptom of IBS as constant toilet habits may lead to dehydration.

**\*Migraines:**

These may range from a mild headache to a full-blown migraine where the sufferer may experience nausea and may need to rest in a darkened room. Besides migraines, cluster headaches may become a problem.

**\*Depression:**

This psychological disorder often associates with FMS. This cycle of prolonged pain may often trigger a period of low mood.

\*Major depression is more serious than a period of low mood, which accompanies FMS.

It is essential to seek professional help with any form of mood change.

\*GP's prescribe most FMS sufferers antidepressant medication as long periods of widespread pain is wearisome and causes most sufferers misery.

**\*Lupus**:

This may be a life-threatening autoimmune disease which sees the body attack its own healthy cells.

\*Lupus patients are easier to diagnose as the initial symptom is a rash across the cheeks and nose, which gets worse in sunlight. This group of patients may also experience joint pains that may or may not cause stiffness, swelling and abnormal movement in the joints.

\*Lupus research is very much in its infancy and researchers are still working to find a connection between this disorder and FMS as both project similar symptoms, apart from the Lupus rash.

\*Both FMS and Lupus may occur together causing sufferers to experience extreme discomfort.

\*A rheumatologist may run several tests to confirm lupus however, a series of blood tests can't diagnose FMS.

**\*Osteoarthritis and Rheumatoid Arthritis:**
These disorders cause the sufferer prolonged excruciating pain, the former being more associated with actual bone pain and the later with the body's joints.

 \*It is not uncommon to have both FMS and either of the two forms of arthritis.

**\*Interstitial cystitis:**
(IC) This bladder condition produces pain and pressure in the bladder region. Inflammation of the bladder wall may cause this disorder.

\*Symptoms may vary from urinary frequency, lower back pain and lower abdominal pain which worsens as the bladder fills and is often mistaken for a urinary tract infection.

\*A GP's may recommend a patient to combine medicine, therapy and lifestyle changes to improve any discomfort from IC.

**\*Temporomandibular disorder:**
This disorder endures the sufferer to extreme pain along with a clicking noise sensed in the muscle which moves the jaw.

**\*Eye Problems:**
Most FMS patients often consider that FMS relates to muscle, tendon and skeletal tissue. They do not consider that FMS may affect our sensory organs, but it takes six main muscles to control eye movements. FMS eye problems are more common than you may think. They produce glitches such as dry eyes, blurred vision or light sensitivity.

**\*Night driving problems:**
A reaction to bright lights and blurred vision may occur, because the eye muscles are not moving as they should.

This may become a permanent problem and sufferers may need to visit an eye infirmary.

**\*Skin rashes:**

These can vary in size and appear anywhere on the body. A rash may cause a crawling sensation on the skin and an itch unrelieved by scratching.

**Temperature intolerance:**

Outside temperatures may affect pain levels, as hot or extreme damp weather can exaggerate symptoms.

\*Temperature sensitivity can play a big role in selecting clothing. What can start out as a cosy comforting sweater on a cold day, can become a baking irritation if the heating is too high. On the other hand, a cool breeze can make you regret wearing a pair of shorts and a T-shirt or light cotton clothing.

\*For those people whom suffer both hot and cold sensitivity, determining what to wear and enduring the consequences of an incorrect choice can be disagreeable, as you either freeze or overheat, or even alternate between the two.

**Endometriosis**:

This condition occurs when the lining of the uterus breaks away and has nowhere to go.

It is a painful condition in which tissue that lines the internal part of the uterus, grows on the outside wall of the uterus.

\*This condition may affect the ovaries and cysts may form. We know these cysts as endometriomas.

\*Symptoms may include painful periods, back and pelvic pain, discomfort during or after sexual intercourse, pain with a bowel movement or urination, infertility, bloating, nausea, heavy cramps, constipation or diarrhoea and bloating.

**\*Periodic limb movement disorder**:
(PLMD) produces repetitive jerking and cramping of the legs during sleep. The repetitive jerking is involuntary.

**\*Anxiety:**
This nervous system disorder accompanies depression, but it may occur from nowhere, with no known cause to trigger an attack.

\*Many patients experience high anxiety, which may trigger a full-blown panic attack. Such episodes may produce heart palpitations, a shortness of breath, flushing and dizziness.

\*A sufferer's blood pressure may drop while an anxiety attack is occurring, and patients may fear they can't get enough air into their lungs and think they will die.

\*Panic attacks are frightening and may cause agoraphobia, an anxiety disorder that causes the sufferer to avoid leaving the home for fear of further anxiety attacks.

**\*Hair loss:**
Thinning of the hair or actual hair loss is common. Medication may be the culprit as many prescription drugs have unwanted side effects.

**\*Muscle tears:**
Tears are common. Many people experience intolerable pain when a tear in any muscle occurs. The rotator cuff is most vulnerable to tear and may strike without cause or reason.

**\*Unexplained bruising**:
 FMS sufferers find themselves clumsier than they were before their diagnosis. Sometimes a slight knock to a limb may go unnoticed, as pain is a common daily occurrence. A minor bump into an article of furniture

may go unnoticed and may be accountable for unexplained marks.

*Fibro fog may be a culprit for bruising, as FMS sufferers struggle with forgetfulness. They may not remember a slight knock or the stubbing of a finger or toe, and then wake up with a nasty bruise.

*Sleep deprivation is another reason for prolonged bruising, because an FMS sufferer lacks restorative sleep and bruises take longer to heal than those of a healthy person and are more noticeable.

**\*Night Sweats:**

Hot flushes and night sweats not associated to pre-or-post menopause may occur which often causes excess sweat and may drench a sufferers clothing.

**Epstein-Barr Virus**:

(EBV) Researchers suspect this viral illness could be a trigger for FMS and CF.

The **Epstein-Barr** herpes virus is from the same family as the chickenpox and cold-sore virus Herpes.

*The virus is more sinister when contracted as an adult but in most cases a complete recovery is possible within a few weeks. Sometimes the virus may reactivate.

*When the virus reactivates, they know it as chronic **Epstein-Barr** Virus Infection.

*People with FMS have a reduced functioning immune system, thus making them more vulnerable to a reactivation of the illness.

*This unpleasant disorder may be a trigger to the onset of FMS.

**Plantar fasciitis:**

*The plantar fascia acts as a shock-absorbing filament supporting the arch in your foot. Tension and stress in this part of the foot may cause small tears in the fascia.

* Repetitive tears cause the fascia to become inflamed.

*This is one of the most common causes of foot pain. It is an inflammation of a band of tissue that connects your heel bone to your toes. It causes a stabbing pain felt worse in the morning but may last for a longer period if you are standing most of the day. The pain may radiate across the inside of your foot or be widespread across both feet. It affects the bottom of the feet and the heels. Sometimes the cause of plantar fasciitis is unknown.

*Steroid injections are helpful in easing the pain associated with this disorder.

**\*Allodynia**:

Allodynia is a hypersensitive reaction to stimuli which results in a pain reaction and comes in three forms:

**Tactile Allodynia,** also called Static Allodynia, causes pain by light touch or pressure. Something as simple as a shower spray, tight clothing, a hug or slight touch may cause unnatural pain.

**Mechanical Allodynia** is movement related. You may experience pain by something touching your skin, such as a bedsheet brushing against you, towelling yourself dry, or putting on clothing.

**Thermal allodynia** is temperature related, and pain occurs with the mildest of temperature change; you may experience your hands and feet burn if they are cold, and ache when they are hot.

**Vitamin D Deficiency:**

At least 25% of FMS sufferers are **Vitamin D** deficient.

*This important vitamin is essential for bone strength, cell growth, neuromuscular health and aids the immune system.

*A lack of this vitamin may cause osteoporosis and high inflammatory markers in your blood.

* A deficiency may explain why FMS sufferers need a higher dose of opioid pain killers than those with the correct balance of vitamin D.

*They relate low vitamin D levels to bone pain, brittleness, muscle pain, muscle weakness, problems with oral membranes and unexplained fatigue.

**B12 Deficiency:**

A deficiency of **Vitamin B12** is common in FMS sufferers. It may present itself as listlessness and fatigue, pale or jaundice skin, pins and needles, dizziness, hair loss, disturbed vision, breathlessness and mood swings.

*You are at risk of developing a deficiency in this vitamin if your body cannot absorb it or you don't get enough **B12** in your food.

**Candida overgrowth:**

Candida is a fungus or yeast overgrowth. A small quantity exists in your intestines along with friendly bacteria. This small quantity causes no harm to the body.

*When overproduced, candida breaks into the wall of the intestines and infiltrates your bloodstream. This causes a host of unpleasant symptoms such as fatigue, digestive issues and pain, and may contribute to brain fog and digestive issues.

**Glossitis and oral problems:**

Tongue and oral problems are common with FMS. Glossitis is an inflammation which causes a sore, red and often swollen tongue. It is a painful condition that makes your tongue appear smooth. The reason this happens is because your taste buds stretch out and disappear.

*You may experience oral symptoms such as mouth ulcers, a burning feeling, or an itching sensation in your mouth.

*Oral thrush may occur after a course of antibiotics, which kills the good bacteria in your gut causing mayhem to the soft oral membranes in your mouth.

**Gastric Intestinal problems:**

Many people with FMS experience gastrointestinal symptoms. Studies have revealed that irritable bowel syndrome, **IBS,** and other **GI** problems coexist with FMS.

*Food intolerances, gas, bloating, excess acid and nausea are commonplace with GI issues.

***GERD, (**gastroesophageal reflux disorder) is higher in patients who have FMS.

*This digestive illness affects the lower oesophagus sphincter, which is a ring of muscle between the oesophagus and stomach. Symptoms may include acid indigestion and heartburn.

***Gastroesophageal reflux** is the return of the stomach's contents back up into the oesophagus.

* **Gastroparesis** is a delayed gastric emptying of the stomach into the bowel. Symptoms may include abdominal bloating, weight loss, nausea and a lack of appetite.

*There are many GI ailments know to coexist with FMS. **IBD** (inflammatory bowel disease) is a good example.

***Crohn's** disease and **Colitis** are typical of IBD's and are debilitating conditions on their own without the added extra of FMS, but these unpleasant illnesses often run side-by-side.

**\*Peripheral Neuropathy:**
Neuropathy is a painful medical condition caused by nerve damage. This disorder may produce tingling, burning and numbness in the hands or feet. It may trigger a weak heavy feeling in the limbs, causing the sufferer to lose their grip and have balance and co-ordination difficulties.

**Pruritus:**
Pruritus is a disorder that many people with FMS experience. It's a constant itch which may affect the quality of your life. It may interrupt your sleep and make life a misery. Prolonged itching and scratching can increase the intensity of the itch possibly leading to skin injury and scarring.

\*Pruritus may be caused by a reaction to certain medications although it has been known to occur without any obvious reason.

\*Unexplained itching must be reported to your GP as severe itching may be contributed to an abnormal liver function.

**\*Fibro Fog:**
Fibro fog is also referred to as brain freeze. Anyone suffering with FMS, have almost certainly experienced memory and concentration problems. You may suffer from poor memory recall, a lack of concentration, forgetfulness, problems pronouncing words, and recalling the names of people and objects. This disorder may worsen with stress, insomnia, medication or overstimulation. It is a debilitating and often embarrassing part of your illness.

FMS causes dysfunction of the muscular, nervous, digestive, immune, reproductive, endocrine, and lymphatic system. There are over 200 additional symptoms to accompany the disorder. I'm sure you've experienced many more coexisting illnesses that have not been included in this chapter. I have covered none of the above disorders in depth. If I've missed details out it is because I am not a medical professional and the information offered results from my research over the years.

During this research I discovered a percentage of children experience widespread pain and coexisting disorders. This was life changing news for me and made perfect sense of my life. My own problems started as a child. I remember burning aches in my limbs on a morning. My diagnosis was growing pains. Do we get pains while we are growing? As children we accept what we are told. I assumed every child experienced pain and my discomfort was accepted as a typical development of youth.

I can't say I was a normal child. While my siblings slept, I used to sleepwalk around the house. I experienced vivid dreams. Because of this restlessness I suffered with fatigue. I became a troublesome youngster. I was always fighting and became problematic throughout my school years. It's a possibility that, if I slept better as a child and my muscles restored themselves, then my younger years may have been different. I may not have suffered from relentless frustration. It's my belief that my journey with FMS began in childhood and, with each stressful event I have experienced, it gathered momentum causing further destruction to an already broken body.

Can you imagine a child experiencing FMS along with these dreadful cohabiting disorders? In the next chapter we will look at how this illness compacts a child life.

# Chapter 3
# Juvenile Fibromyalgia Syndrome (JFS)

### Growing pain vs JFS

It is debatable if growing pains exist. After engaging in several debates on the subject I researched the topic and found that if a child becomes active and uses various muscles, then they will experience pain until the muscles involved become accustomed to working.

These aches and pains may last a few days or longer and a doctor may attribute them to growing pains. However, if a child experiences widespread pain with no cause or reason and the pain is long lasting then it should ring alarm bells.

If growing pains exist, it would suggest that every child on the planet experiencing a growth spurt would be in agony. Is this realistic? I don't think so.

There is a huge difference between **Juvenile Fibromyalgia Syndrome** and childhood aches and pains. One complaint is bearable and the other is intolerable. It can render a child immobile.

Those children who receive a diagnosis of growing pains are the minority who end up with FMS in adulthood or JFS in adolescence.

When a child complains of obscure symptoms, it may be difficult to find the root cause of the problem. Children may complain of tiredness, sleeping problems or suffer from aches and pains in various parts of their bodies. This can raise concerns for parents. It is easy for a doctor to overlook JFS as it's more common in adults. One of the main symptoms are sore areas on or around the muscles. These are trigger points. To find these points the examining doctor will press with his/her thumb on eighteen areas. To fit the criteria a child only needs to experience pain in at least three specific points. A GP will ask if the aches and pains have been ongoing for at least three months or more. This may show the GP that further investigations require his/her attention, and they ought to test for underlying disorders.

## JFS Facts
*FMS affects children despite the common misconception it's an age-related disease JFS is becoming more recognisable in childhood. The medical profession calls it "Juvenile Fibromyalgia Syndrome" (JFS).

*It is more common in female children, and they diagnose most children around the age of thirteen to fifteen. Between 1% and 7% of children in the USA have JFS, or similar conditions. The percentage for the UK is unknown at present.

*GP's observing children who present joint pains are much more likely to consider a Vitamin D deficiency, or diagnose the infamous condition known as growing pains.

*Dealing with chronic pain can be tough for children, since other people may perceive them as being healthy. It's common for children with JFS to experience depression or become anxious. They may find it hard to cope at school and just stay home when they're not well.

*One of the main reasons JFS can be so frustrating for children is that its symptoms often compound one another. For example, the pain experienced as part of the disorder, makes it problematic to sleep. When children can't sleep, they tire during the day. It becomes a vicious cycle that most children find difficult to break.

*Teenagers with the disorder may find it difficult making friends, and become unpopular, because of the stigma often attached to their condition.

*JFS does not cause harm to your child's body tissue or organs.

*There's no evidence that JFS will affect your child's lifespan.

*There is no test which can show if your child will develop JFS.

*JFS and CFS present themselves together.

*You can support your child's health. by ensuring they eat a balanced, healthy diet.

*Children often cope better with pain than adults.

*Around nine out of ten JFS child patients are female

*JFS is uncommon in children younger than four.

*It is more difficult to receive a diagnosis for a child.

### JFS Symptoms

*Children may complain of soreness in one part of the body which may begin in the limbs and move to other areas.

*Children describe pain in different ways. They may say they are aching or experiencing pain in their arms and legs. The location and intensity of pain varies from one child to another. It's often described as a dull ache in the muscles of the arms, legs, back and neck. Most children complain of "burning", "throbbing", or "shooting" pains, or experience pain which radiates outward from specific parts of their body.

*Children may have sleep difficulties such as sleepwalking or restlessness. They may be a light sleeper and wake up tired and lethargic.

*They appear to show little enthusiasm and cannot join in games with friends or at school.

*Teenagers often display symptoms of anxiety and depression.

*Stomach aches are common as younger children often find it difficult to explain where the pain radiates.

*Forgetfulness, stumbling, or being clumsy is another sign of JFS.

*Restless Leg Syndrome. A child may be fidgety when their legs are uncomfortable, and they may need to move them often.

*A child cannot join in games and activities because of fatigue.

*JFS may centre pain in muscles and ligaments or be more widespread.

*The pain can range from a dull ache to a stabbing pain along with tingling or numbness.

*A child may experience nausea and discomfort from pain.

Parents may worry they could have prevented their child's JFS or looked for ways to make sure it doesn't develop in any of their other children; but there's no known way to stop it from occurring.

## A Diagnosis

*The first port of call is a GP. He/she examines the child and refers them to a team of specialists such as a paediatric rheumatologist, and a psychologist if his/her opinion is swaying towards JFS.

*A GP is likely to make a first diagnosis of growing pains.

*Besides a physical examination, your doctor will ask if the child has sleeping problems and if they have experienced low moods.

*JFS can be harder to diagnose in children because it's much more common in adults. As with adults, no cure for JFS is available, and treatments will involve trial and error.

*While no lab test may confirm a diagnosis of JFS, your doctor may want to rule out other conditions, such as **Juvenile Arthritis**, which presents similar symptoms.

*A GP will consider blood tests. These may include a complete blood count and a thyroid test

*GP's are reticent to start drugs at a young age, knowing most medicines prescribed to JFS patients are addictive.

## Coping Strategies

Coping Strategies, such as those listed below may help your child endure the negative side of JFS. They are essential to the young sufferer of JFS, who must try to stay positive, and learn to adapt to their disorder.

*Assure your child there are ways to improve their lifestyle.

*Basic methods of easing the symptoms of JFS may include muscle relaxation and stress-relieving techniques such as deep breathing or visualisation.

*Children with the condition who stay active may experience less pain, less social isolation and less depression.

*Getting enough sleep is one of the most effective ways to treat JFS. It's a good idea to eliminate caffeine, sodas and snacks right before bedtime. Children should go to bed and rise at the same time each day. Limit napping during the daytime.

* Find activities that may help distract your child from their JFS symptoms.

*Sessions with a specialised paediatric physiotherapist and massage can ease muscle soreness that children with the disorder often experience.

*Regular exercise may increase your child's pain at first, but exercise can ease the symptoms of JFS in the long run.

*Research has proven your child may show improvement from stretching and relaxation exercises.

We don't know why children contract JFS, but researchers assume both genetic and environmental factors are at fault.

It's important to remember JFS just happens and there's nothing you could do to prevent its onset.

## Childhood JFMS Stories

### Alisa Rose

Alisa is ten years old; she is a JFS warrior. Her short life has been fraught with an illness from the age of three. Her problems began after a diagnosis of **Vaginal Lichen Sclerosus**. It's a rare condition affecting the skin between the vagina and anus. The skin tissue is paper thin and may tear easy. This is a traumatic disease which affects post-menopausal women. Besides this unpleasant condition Alicia has JFS.

### Charlotte C

My daughter Alisa 10 years old sufferers from a condition which produces debilitating symptoms, along with JFS.

The following notes are from a diary I kept during Alisa's hospital appointments, from October 2018 to May 2019.

**Alisa's Health Diary**

**1ˢᵗ October 2018:** I took Alisa to hospital. She has double vision and widespread aches and pains. The doctors gave us a further appointment.

**9ᵗʰ November 2018:** Alisa still had problems with her vision. The hospital advised eye exercises and a further appointment for a review.

**15ᵗʰ December 2018:** Alisa can't focus well, and her eyes are turning inwards. We have noticed no positive change in her vision. The hospital arranged for a four-month review.

**27ᵗʰ January 2019:** The skin between Alisa's vagina and anus has torn. They have admitted her onto the children's ward.

Alisa is wheelchair bound. The school have put risk assessments in place for her to attend school.

**25ᵗʰ February 2019:** Alisa has been to the hospital since 7.15pm. Her right leg is numb, she has pins and needles from her knee to her toes. She cannot bear weight on her leg and has no mobility. The doctors are unsure what is causing the problem and they are organising a hip x-ray. They have taken blood samples. This is confusing, and I am worried.

**26thFebruary 2019:** A doctor admitted Alisa onto the children's ward. No one can explain why she is experiencing these alarming symptoms.

They are reluctant to X-ray the full leg because of radiation. They have sent her home with medication and I am to bring her back on Thursday. We arrived home after a long day and night. but they have told us to return if the problem deteriorates.

**28thFebruary2019:** Alisa has undergone more physical tests. There have been no scans or x-rays up to now. The doctors can't conclude or diagnose what may cause this problem. Two neurology doctors have spoken to an orthopaedic specialist. I should receive answers soon. I am assuming they will give my daughter a scan. She's admitted to the ward again. I returned home for a while and Mum stayed at the hospital. Alisa went for an x-ray. We will know more tomorrow when a senior orthopaedic doctor will talk to us in the morning.

**1st March 2019:** A long night in the hospital with Alisa again. They have informed me they will repeat blood tests and do another X-ray and an MRI scan.

**8th March 2019:** We have been for an MRI scan. It's now a waiting game for the results and to speak with her consultant.

**1st April 2019:** Alisa is back at the hospital for her vision review, which has not improved. This continues to alarm me. Pins and needles are spreading to her arms so, the specialist, has suggested she receives a head scan.

**10th April 2019:** Alisa is wheelchair bound. The school have put risk assessments in place for her to attend school.

**15th April:** Physiotherapy is in place and Alisa is more mobile.

**1st May 2019:** Alisa is mobile for the first time since the 25th February.

**26th May2019:** We are back at the hospital talking to a specialist. The test results are back and reveal nothing sinister.

After a thorough examination the specialist looked at me and said, "You must know my diagnosis. Your daughter has **Juvenile Fibromyalgia Syndrome**".

My heart sank, as a sufferer myself, I know what my daughter's future entails. Alisa struggles to sleep, she wakes each morning in pain. I believe she is in shock at her diagnosis of JFMS. She has seen how this illness has affected my life. She is worried for her future, as am I.

I know first-hand how debilitating this cruel illness affects an adult. It is unjust my daughter should endure this at a young age. It's so sad that my daughter must cope with two debilitating disorders for the rest of her life, but I will do my utmost to keep her mind frame positive.

## Annabel D, aged 16

At fourteen, after a period of illness, I received a diagnosis of glandular fever along with a viral infection. This cost me three months leave of absence from school. During this period, I became so ill I only left the house to visit my GP. When my body showed no sign of recovering, they ordered blood tests to rule out sinister illnesses. My results came back normal, and the GP suggested I had CFS. I can't say I experienced much pain apart from the odd nagging ache in my chest but the fatigue I endured became extreme.

On my return to school the teachers reduced my timetable to three days a week, but even on a short school week I returned home to sleep. My parents became alarmed at the excessive time I spent lounging around and sleeping. The fatigue wiped me out and I became incapable of performing any small task. My friends assumed I was lazy by refusing to go places with them, and the school I attended was unhappy that my attendance has dropped. No one understood my problems and I became depressed. Friends disappeared and I felt lonely and abandoned.

My life became a daily chore of school eat, sleep and repeat. Everything changed two months later when I experienced migraines, extreme chest pains and picked up every bug going. Whatever this illness was it was giving me a hard time. I was sinking in quicksand and couldn't pull myself free. I often forgot things and experienced confusion. My concentration disappeared and dizziness became the bane of my life. At aged fourteen my life had crumbled.

My vision became affected, my eyes became swollen and to add further misery to my sad life, I developed painful mouth ulcers. This resulted in a further three months absence from school.

Out of concern my parents took me back to the GP. He took more bloods which produced negative results. The doctor discussed my singular symptoms instead of looking at the bigger picture. It became a frustrating and depressing time. Not long after this gloomy period my body projected extreme widespread pain which I can only describe as electric shocks. I cried bitter tears for my unjust life.

One year later my doctor suggested my pain was comparable to JFS and referred me to a muscular skeletal clinic. The clinic refused to treat me because at aged sixteen they considered me a child. They passed me on to general paediatrics who diagnosed JFS and CFS, and they referred me to an adult clinic. The hospital refused the referral because I didn't fit the criteria age wise. It is unbelievable that I am now waiting for an appointment back to general paediatrics My mind is in turmoil and my parents worry for my future.

I have every symptom of JFS and several coexisting disorders along with a definite diagnosis, yet, I am in limbo because of my age. The NHS has failed me. I am sixteen years old suffering with JFS, yet no department will accept me.

In two years, my life has changed beyond measure I should be enjoying myself by going shopping and hanging out with friends. Instead I live a life with an invisible disease that shows me no mercy.

I have accepted my illness and have overcome the bitterness and frustration I first experienced when my illness began. I only hope they change the rules on the age they diagnose a child.

Paediatrics have informed me that different health authorities diagnose children younger than myself. This service should be available across the UK and not in different catchment areas.

JFS is real and can be as debilitating for a child as it is an adult. We know this illness is extreme, but does it progress? In the next chapter we will examine the stages of FMS from two different points of view.

# Chapter 4
# **The 7 Stages of Fibromyalgia**

FMS condemns you to a life of suffering and pain. It is unfortunate that for most sufferers, the longer you have this illness the worse the symptoms become. This doesn't offer much hope to those diagnosed, but it's a fact.

The American College of Rheumatology suggest seven stages of FMS exist, each one progressing. For example, as a child I hoped my supposed growing pains improved in adulthood, but I was wrong. They became worse with time and age. Each phase became more difficult to endure. My body deteriorated at each distinct period.

Below, I present you with what I consider the seven stages of FMS. I came to this conclusion after taking extensive notes from my journey with FMS and compared the data I had accumulated from friends who have endured this illness for many years.

If you experience any symptoms you may think resonates with FMS, seek medical advice early to get the correct treatment plan.

### Stage one

There are four main symptoms which include widespread pain, insomnia, fatigue and depression. It begins with pain and fatigue. At this stage it's endurable, but it could become problematic. It does not prevent you from working or doing chores such as cleaning up or going for shopping, you may even enjoy the occasional night out. At this stage regardless of the aches and fatigue you can still manage your day but because of pain and occasional tiredness you suspect something is wrong with your body. Hence, you research and look for answers. You may visit the doctor complaining of vague symptoms but prepare yourself for his/her scepticism. There are many medical professionals who are unsympathetic when a patient presents widespread pain. Most medical professionals still lack knowledge and expertise to diagnose FMS. Distinct health authorities differ in treatments, referrals or diagnosing. Much depends which part of the country you live. At this point if you are unhappy with your GP, I suggest you change to a different practice. The sooner you find a health care professional who can offer you a care plan with the correct treatments, the more helpful it may be to your overall health.

You may take over-the-counter medication for bouts of aches, pain and fatigue which may not be much of a problem at this stage. Listen to your body and don't tag any troublesome symptoms as age related or class them as general aches and pain from working.

**Stage two**
At stage two the pain intensifies, and a doctor may prescribe anti-inflammatory drugs. These may work for a short while, but after a few months they appear to grant little relief. Pain may become constant and experienced every day. You may suffer unrefreshing sleep along with bouts of insomnia. This results in further fatigue. Our sleep pattern falls into four stages and because you do not get enough stage four sleep, which regenerates body and muscle tissue, you may find yourself in a cycle

of widespread pain, and CFS caused by a lack of restorative sleep. You may wake up exhausted. It's an unnatural weariness and is not the same as ordinary tiredness. Exhaustion can't get better with rest or sleep; it affects your ability to get on and enjoy your life. You may need stronger pain relief and your doctor will send you for medical tests, but the results may come back normal. The doctor may be unsympathetic to FMS patients and the diagnosis itself. Regardless of your increased pain and fatigue, you may still be in work and socialise on occasions. Enjoy this time for as long as you are able.

**Stage three**
At this stage the pain and fatigue are constant. They both devour your strength and energy, forcing you to spend several days in bed. You try to avoid contact with people and as a result you lose friends. You may not answer the phone, respond to emails, or letters. You may even stop sending birthday or Christmas cards. A lack of enthusiasm engulfs you and low moods may become a regular occurrence. A constant tiredness and lack of sleep affects your strength and energy all day every day. You worry over everything. Finance may become a huge problem if you leave work and go onto benefits. If you are the main bread winner in the house, this can be daunting. At this stage you should seek advice from the **Citizens Advice Bureau**, (CAB) who can help with an application for Personal Independent Payments. (PIPS). You may apply for **PIPS** if you are still working. CAB are helpful and can offer information on your rights to other benefits. Many people are unaware of what they can claim and where to go for help. A rheumatologist may diagnose you with FMS and you now join the

millions of people classed as disabled. I should point out that not everyone gets to see a rheumatologist. It's important to emphasis each symptom to your GP, as many won't or don't refer to other health services.

This stage may go on for a long period, maybe even years

**Stage four**

Here, you experience a blend of unrelenting physical and emotional stress. My experience, and that of others is you just can't stay in bed, as other responsibilities take priority and you may not have anyone to help. You may have to drag yourself up to feed the kids, get them dressed, take them to school and complete household chores. You may spend the rest of your day laying and sleeping on the sofa.

There will be few days whereby your energy levels increase. On, these days you can get things done and enjoy this newfound energy, but you may overdo things which results in further pain and fatigue for the next few days. Your social life goes up in flames as your friends plan events without you. They know you will refuse invitations, so the invites stop altogether.

Family members may become irritated because you stay in bed most of the time. They may even resent you for this and brand you lazy. People around you get angry at your lack of action and become dismissive of any explanation. This could be because in your earlier stages of FMS, you could still get things done. They assume you are using your illness as an excuse to be idle. In effect, they have given up on you which can isolate you further.

## Stage five

You have either given up work or lost your job through constant sick leave.

You no longer have the energy to pursue your dreams and aspirations, and basic hygiene tasks become a huge chore. You may need help with the intimate actions of washing and drying.

Microwave or ready-made meals are easier and more convenient. Your new friends are FMS sufferers and at this stage you may need a mobility aid such as a wheelchair, a mobility scooter, or a push along shopping trolley. If you are lucky a walking stick may be the only mobility aid you need. You may need extra aids to help with hygiene. These may include a shower chair, a long-handled sponge, or a bath bar.

Most people at this stage long for family support and understanding, but not everyone will appreciate the reality of your illness.

## Stage six

You no longer have the energy to do a simple task, getting out of bed, or bathing. It drains you of the little energy you hold. Gone are the days when you took daily showers and attended to your hair. These tasks are limited to once or twice a week. Anti-inflammatory drugs or painkillers become addictive because of continued use. The doctor may have prescribed stronger pain medication such as morphine, and the side effects of these drugs can produce an adverse reaction to your body and internal organs.

By now, several specialists have diagnosed you with other co-morbidities and to top things off, FMS throws every symptom it can your way, making your life a misery.

You can't do much on your own and assume you are a burden to your loved ones. You have no confidence or self-worth. Life is not rosy!

**Stage seven**
This final stage is acceptance and you look for alternative forms of treatment. Acceptance does not mean you surrender, it means, you face this illness from a new perspective. You no longer view yourself as worthless and can cope better with pain. You note the triggers which begin a flare and your knowledge on FMS is vast. Life is painful, but you accept your illness and make the most of every day. Your family may laugh at the funny things which occur when fibro fog strikes. You may use the support offered on social media such as FMS groups and forums. The best group I have found online is FIBROMYALGIA AND CHRONIC ILLNESS UK FAMILY. They offer a listening ear, support and friendship. Someone is always available for a chat, even during the long hours of insomnia.
Regardless of which stage you are at on your FMS journey it won't kill you. You may think you live a miserable life, because you cannot do the activities that were once possible, but life can be worth living once you accept your limitations.

Depression may strike at any stage and often exaggerates your symptoms. Once you receive a diagnosis there's little you can do, It's a lifelong condition. One piece of advice is to find strategies to cope and groups that offer advice. FMS is a multi-faceted illness One of the worst side effects is short term memory loss. Learn to laugh at the mistakes you make while having a fibro fog moment. Find people online, with the same diagnosis as yourself, and you may even make lifelong FMS friends.

I and many others do not allow this constant wretched illness to define who we are. I hope you follow our lead. You can still enjoy a quality of life by finding a happy medium.

You may skip one of these stages or stay at one stage for a long period. No two people are alike, but for most people who suffer with FMS, their condition worsens.

## **A Personal Stage Account from the Internet**

Those who stick to the medical development of the disease may find many accounts available that give personal experiences of individuals interpretation of FMS stages, with perhaps, Angela Wise's 2014 piece being one of the most revered.

Wise depicts the seven stages of her FMS in terms of its increase in severity and how it affected her life.

**1** The sufferer experiences additional pain and discomfort and knows that something isn't right, but it's not enough to derail daily life.

**2** Wise suggests that this stage involves a great deal of pain you may receive a diagnosis and although both the expected levels of pain and fatigue have begun, analgesia (pain relief) is useful and life goes on.

**3** She suggests a sufferer will withdraw from social and family activities, and other than going to work, they are likely to need extra rest.

**4** This stage will see a sufferer isolated and alone as friends will have stopped offering invites to activities, pain will be present most of the time and the occasional few good days are welcome.

**5** In this stage, Wise suggests that sufferers consider that they have a permanent disability and may have to quit work.

**6** FMS is a way of life. Pain and fatigue have taken total control and sufferers are pretty much housebound. Attempts to live a regular life to reduce feelings of guilt and being a burden, is a struggle, and the routine people once took for granted have vanished.

**7** Wise suggests this is the stage of acceptance, where the sufferer accepts the way of life, or what remains of it.

If we compare both accounts you will find they are similar in the way both sufferers, and the medical professionals describe the progress of FMS

# Chapter 5
# **Let's Talk Medication**

A cure is unavailable for FMS at this time. The best you may hope for is a good medication regime, to treat pain and other coexisting symptoms. We each differ in our tolerances to medications, and what may be helpful to one person may not be, to another. I do not intend this chapter to direct you for self-treatment. A GP will decide what's best for you, he/she will play an important role in your treatment and care according to which treatments are available, via your medical health authority.

There are several horror stories which hit the media when vital medication was unavailable for people with cancer because of their catchment zone. The same rule applies to any prescribed medications including CBD oil.

GP's will prescribe CBD oil for various illnesses, but it's a postcode lottery and not every doctor can or will do this. Some GP's are prescribing this oil for chronic pain and epilepsy, but many are reluctant in handing out this natural treatment. If you wish to follow a natural approach, CBD is available via the internet or at your local health store, but try to find a reliable, trusted source.

All medication comes with adverse effects. If we took the time to read the side effects listed in the information leaflet, I doubt if we would take any kind of prescribed drugs. If you do experience side effects of any medication, stop them at once and contact your GP.

Most prescription drugs offered to FMS patients are habit forming but what other alternative do you have when you require some quality pain free living?

## Medications

Simple painkillers accessible over the counter from a pharmacy, such as **Paracetamol**, **Ibuprofen**, and Co-Codamol can sometimes help give relief associated with general aches and pains, but these drugs have their own set of side-effects and prolonged use can cause damage to the body. For instance, **Ibuprofen,** is likely to exacerbate IBS, so make sure you read the manufacturer's instructions on any pharmacy medicine you buy.

Over-the-counter painkillers are not effective for constant widespread pain, so you may need stronger medications such as **Codeine Phosphate** or **Tramadol** Please note these painkillers can be addictive, and their effectiveness diminishes over time with repeated usage, so the dosage may need increasing.

Let us look at some known drugs prescribed for FMS sufferers

### *Amitriptyline:

GP's often prescribe **Amitriptyline** for FMS patients. While they know this medication as an antidepressant, it also treats migraines, insomnia, anxiety and FMS. As with most drugs this medicine causes side effects, and the most noted is weight gain, excessive perspiring and hair thinning.

Amitriptyline alters the level of hormones in our body, leading to increased appetite and cravings, which make some people susceptible to storing fat. Carb cravings are heightened by this drug. Eating carbs in excess creates fat storage and weight gain, which may lead to depression in those people concerned about body image.

## Pregabalin and Gabapentin:

Their main use of these drugs is for epilepsy, but research has shown that they may improve pain associated with FMS They both prevent sensitive nerves from sending pain signals to the brain, these medicines curb your pain, aid fatigue and help insomnia, but the side effects noted are weight gain, oedema (swelling of hands and feet), dizziness, drowsiness and blurred vision.

## Antipsychotics

Antipsychotic medicines, also called Neuroleptics, helps relieve long-term pain. Several studies have shown that these medications may help conditions like FMS.

## Antidepressants:

Anti-depressants boost the levels of chemicals that carry communications to and from the brain, otherwise known as neurotransmitters. Low levels of these chemicals may be a causative factor in FMS. The medical community suggest that antidepressant medication can be effective in treating FMS and it's believed that it may relieve pain for some people with the disorder. However, despite their effectiveness, antidepressants may cause several unwanted side effects including nausea, a dry mouth, drowsiness, agitation, shakiness or anxiety, dizziness, weight gain and constipation.

There are many types of anti-depressants and you GP will prescribe them on the severity of your symptoms. They may prescribe you one of the following drugs. These are the most common used medications for depression.
*Fluoxetine (Prozac)
*Duloxetine
*Paroxetine
*Venlafaxine
This list is by no means complete, and your GP may try you on several medications before you find one that is suitable. This is because every medication available, even an over-the-counter drug, comes with its own collection of side effects. It may take you several attempts trying different medications until you find one which agrees with you.

### Sleep Medications:

Improving sleep is an important part of assisting FMS. A chronic lack of sleep can affect your overall health and immune system. If you can control your quality of sleep it may help concentration and fatigue.
Suffers of muscle stiffness or spasms (when the muscles contract) may receive a prescription for a muscle relaxant, such as **Diazepam**. These types of medicines may help you sleep better, because of their sedative (sleep-inducing) effect.
**\*Diazepam:** Is both a sedative and muscle relaxant. Most GP's are reluctant to prescribe these as they are

habit forming, and doctors recommend you don't drive or use machinery while taking this medication, which may be problematic for those who drive. This drug is useful in treating muscle spasticity (a painful condition where the muscles contract). They are excellent when used as a muscle relaxer. While they don't stop nerve endings from emitting unnecessary pain signals, they slow the process down and have the added benefit of a sedative effect caused from anxiety. Most doctors refuse to add these in your treatment regime or only offer them as a short-term solution.

**\*Temazepam:** They use this common medicine to treat insomnia, and it is often as a relaxant before a surgical procedure. These tablets are addictive, so doctors refuse to prescribe it for long term use. The recommended time for taking these drugs are ten days, because of their habit-forming quality.

**\*Zopiclone:** This medicine helps you fall asleep and stops you waking up during the night. It takes around one hour to work efficiently. The side effects are a metallic taste, or dryness in your mouth.

**\*Mirtazapine:** This has a sedative effect and is an excellent to aid sleep. It has side effects, one of these being weight gain regardless of diet. My regime of medication includes Mirtazapine. My GP prescribed this for both depression and insomnia. It works well, but the side effects are unwelcome.

**Opioids:**
This type of medication blocks pain messages sent from the body, through the spinal cord to the brain. While they can effectively relieve widespread pain, opioids are highly addictive when taken long term.

*There are several types of prescribed opioids. Codeine, Fentanyl, Oxycodone and Morphine are commonly used for FMS. These are only available via a GP.

*Opioids can be part of an effective pain management plan, but to help avoid side effects and risk of addiction only take the prescribed amount.

*A common reaction from this medicine may include nausea, tiredness and constipation. If taken long term liver or bowel damage could occur.

*Take only as directed by your GP and read the information leaflet provided.

Again, this medication list is not complete. I have only listed the most common medications prescribed.

Anyone suffering with FMS is sure to be taking an assortment of medications which may have side effects, and most are addictive, so what choice does that leave a sufferer?

We take medication to help with our daily pain and other co-morbidities, and then, we endure more problems with adverse reactions. We are obligated to take into consideration pain, medication, side effect and/or addiction.

It's a game we can't win, as coexisting disorders invade our body, and this increases the amount of prescription drugs we take, so more people are seeking a holistic approach to managing their pain.

## Self Help

We often find people with FMS to have low levels of vitamin D, and as low vitamin D levels affect the ability of bones to absorb calcium, it could lead to a reduction in bone density, which could worsen pain.

*An increase in Vitamin D in rich food such as leafy greens, oranges, and an increase in calcium via consumption of dairy produce, could prove helpful, but extra supplements may be a necessary step.

*Studies have shown alcohol consumption is fine in moderation, with light to moderate, alcohol drinkers having a better quality of life. They suffer less severe symptoms than non-drinkers. Moderate suggests, between three and five alcoholic drinks per week, but not a full bottle in one day. The chance to overindulge would be nice, but medication makes alcohol a problem. You can still enjoy a drink in moderation, I love nothing better than quiet time with a nice glass of Merlot

*Caffeine may make you more alert and aids fibro fog, but it can make sleeping difficult. Four or more cups of caffeinated drinks per day may increase FMS pain, so switch to decaf. I found the switch over easy and noticed no change in the taste of my coffee.

*A lot of FMS sufferers have changed to a clean eating programme in the hope it improves their overall health. A healthful diet not only benefits your physical self, it improves mental health. The nutrients such as vitamin B-6 help make dopamine, a chemical involved in feeling pleasure. Omega-3 fatty acids are a good support for mental health, while a deficiency leads to depression. Clean eating is cutting out processed food and sugars. This is not always possible. Not everyone can't afford to buy fresh ingredients daily, or even get out of the house to buy them. I rely on someone else cooking my meals, and I appreciate that support. I eat what they prepare for me. Those who have a family and a home to

care for without the added pressure of FMS, may find this clean eating diet or any diet impossible.

## Alternative Therapies

More people are turning to complementary or alternative treatments and therapies to ease their symptoms These treatments are becoming more popular with FMS patients.

I have tried most of the treatments mentioned. As suggested previously, we differ in our likes and dislikes, should you choose to try the natural route. I am sure you may find a favourite treatment to help with your overall well-being.

**Acupuncture:** This Chinese medical practice is a popular treatment. It relieves pain by the insertion fine needles placed into pressure points around the body. It's a painless procedure and is effective in treating widespread or localised pain

**\*Reflexology:** Reflexology involves a therapist applying pressure to the soles of your feet with specific hand techniques, without oil or lotions. I found it amazing for my tired and painful feet, when the technician has finished the treatment, they offer you a soothing foot massage.

**\*Aromatherapy:** My favourite relaxation treatment is aromatherapy. It uses aromatic materials, including essential oils and other compounds to produce blends of oil, which improves your psychological and physical well-being.

Essential oils don't just add aromas to the room, they offer many health benefits for the household. Placing oils in a diffuser allows various aromas to fill a room with your favourite fragrance.

Applying balms and lotions may be the most effective way to treat pain, but a diffuser can enhance the effect. Both oils and diffusers are inexpensive and are worth trying.

**\*Swedish Massage:** This massage technique works the soft tissues of the body by kneading, friction, effleurage and tapping. It's said to improve circulation, ease muscular tension and promote relaxation.

**\*Meditation:** We use meditation to focus on the present moment. It can help to quiet your mind whilst relaxing your muscles. There are many apps or recordings free on the Internet.

**\*Mindfulness:** This is knowing and being in tune with our bodies both inside and outside of ourselves. It's a way of understanding how our thoughts can influence our emotions and subsequent behaviour. Paying more attention to the present moment and your own thoughts and feelings can improve your mental wellbeing.

There is very little scientific evidence that such treatments help FMS symptoms in the long term, but people find that therapies can help them relax and de-destress, permitting them to cope with their condition better.

Most GP surgeries have a well-being clinic in their practice, which is worth pursuing. For example, my GP's practice offers a clinic for dietary advice, relaxation classes and group therapy for patients with mental health, but not every health authority offer these services. It's worth enquiring at your own surgery to see what's on offer.

I have only mentioned a few of the medication and therapies available. Many more are accessible. Try your local college, they usually offer treatments at a reduced price for students to practice their techniques

# Chapter 6
# **Educating Family**

*Communication matters in a relationship where one partner is a sufferer of FMS*

Many misconceptions exist on what causes FMS, its symptoms and how to treat it. This illness can frustrate family members if they are unaware of how your disorder limits you. Often those with a diagnosis of FMS won't want to appear as a "complainer" or a "burden to others". Many sufferers will try to put on a happy face, hide their pain and get on with their lives. This is a foolish step, as your family needs to understand your limitations. They deserve to know how you are feeling daily and what kinds of things might make your symptoms worse.

It's problematic for somebody who doesn't have FMS or any form of invisible illness such as chronic pain to envisage what living with the disorder entails, but they need to know, so they may understand your needs.

As much as you may struggle to come to terms with your condition or a new diagnosis of FMS, your family and friends will find it difficult too. They may be unaware on what is happening in your life and how it affects you. The more facts you tell your family the more supportive and understanding they might be.

FMS sufferers often miss out on family events and celebrations. It's no fun being among a group of people who are drinking, singing, dancing and having fun, while you are in extreme pain and discomfort. Often excuses are made to evade such gatherings; but missed activities are not just tough on the sufferer, they are hard on everybody involved. Friends and family assume you don't wish to mix and often find you unsociable. This is because they are not aware of FMS facts and how the disorder impacts your life.

It's never easy to see a loved one in pain. Education is important, both for yourself and for those sharing your life. If you have problems explaining the impact of FMS, the following information should help you clarify your disorder. Better still get your family reading this chapter.

### To My Family

*My illness is real. It is invisible and because of this you may view me as exaggerating my symptoms. I can assure you I experience pain every day. Most days the pain is present but bearable. Other days I am unproductive because of excruciating agony.

*My body produces influenza symptoms without the runny nose, cough or sneezes. I ache twenty-four hours a day.

*Fatigue zaps my energy. When this occurs, I am a run-down battery, zero energy, no oomph and no zest for life.

*You may perceive me as miserable. I can assure you I am tired and worn out. This is because my body does not get restorative sleep. I go to bed exhausted and wake up exhausted.

*I am trying to work through the pain to live as normal as I can.

*Planning future events is impossible. I don't know from one day to the next how my body may react.

*My body works like a pre-paid electric meter. I may start the day with £10 in the meter and when the money runs out, my energy stops.

*Trying to live a productive life is difficult for me. Please understand my limitations.

*If you assume, I am ignoring you; I am not. fibro fog plays havoc with my mind. If too many people talk at once, I may experience a sensory overload and walk out of the room. By doing this I am preventing an anxiety attack which is an unpleasant experience.

*My medication may make me drowsy, and when this happens, I need to nap. This is out of my control.

*I may complain of shoulder pain, restless legs, pins and needles in my limbs, insomnia, widespread pain or migraine; these are facets of the same disease. This does not define me a hypochondriac.

*Fibromyalgia has many facades and each day I may experience a new symptom.

*If I wander during the night, I do so to allow you undisturbed sleep.

*I always have doctor appointments, please have patience with me. I am living life the best I can, with an illness that is trying to defeat me.

*Please don't think I am lazy. My illness produces real symptoms.

* Will you take a few minutes to research FMS? Try Google It will lead you to several sites dedicated to FMS such as **NHS Choices** and **Fibromyalgia Action UK**. You may then understand my frustrations.

*Remind me often that stopping is not failing. Your reassurance will comfort me.

*Little things are meaningful. Run me a bath or put my wheat bag in the microwave to show me you care. This illness isolates me I need to feel loved, not feel alone.

*There may be days when I don't wish to talk, give me the space to gather my thoughts.

* When depression strikes, remind me I have so much to live for.

*I am still the same person as I once was, I don't want sympathy I want your understanding.

* Help me finds solutions to my many coexisting illnesses on the days I am too weary to do this myself.

*Have patience when I become angry and frustrated at my illness. It is not my intension to be miserable, I am in a constant battle with my body.

*I have come to terms with my illness and its array of symptoms. Can you please accept me as I am now?

*There are days when I am fragile both in body and mind, hug me when I cry and offer me your support.

* On the days I can't get out of bed bring me a hot drink or lay beside me and talk a while.

I hope the information will provide your family with some understanding as to how your illness affects you, but be aware, there are those who will think you are healthy because your outward appearance does not show the internal chaos raging inside your body.

Never make excuses for yourself You have a debilitating condition that, currently is incurable. As suggested, FMS is not an illness that will kill you, although it will make your life unbearable. No one should ever judge you. Until someone has walked a day in your shoes, they could never imagine the pain and distress you endure on an upside-down day. Hold you head high. You are an FMS warrior, fighting pain the best way you can.

# Chapter 7
# Top Tips from FMS Sufferers

When FMS pain strikes, it may be difficult to find something suitable to help the debilitating symptoms. The following tips and self-help suggestions are from people diagnosed with FMS. They each suggest a coping mechanism; in the hope the reader may find something of use. We each differ in varying degrees to treatments, medications or FMS advice. What one person may find useful another may not. It is my hope you find a beneficial new tip which may offer you support on your FMS journey. One simple piece of advice from another sufferer may limit the amount of prescription medication you use, which is worth bearing in mind.

I have always loved natural remedies, but I also rely on several prescription medications While searching for a natural approach to aid chronic pain and reduce my opioid intake, I stumbled upon a product called '**Pain Slayer.**'

The woody undertones, clean herbal scents and the healing properties of this balm impressed me. Within a short time of using this natural product my pain diminished; therefore, I nominate this as the 'number one tip' for anyone enduring nagging FMS pain. I am not affiliated with the company, so my review is unbiased.

The **Motorbikers Cosmetic Company** use natural, organic, sustainable oils to produce a wide range of products aimed to help FMS sufferers worldwide.

Each item produced is free from harmful parabens, pesticides, GMO's (genetically modified organisms) and are none animal derived Their wide range of healing products offer you a holistic approach to managing pain and may lessen the need for pharmaceutical drugs.

The company manufactures their products in the UK and ship out orders the following day. Your package arrives within a short time by Royal Mail. **Migraines**, **CFS**, **pain** and **insomnia**, may become more manageable by using M.C.C. merchandise. This company is an asset to FMS sufferers. I have listed their contact details in a further chapter.

It is my belief any coping mechanism is invaluable to FMS sufferers therefore; I offer my gratitude to everyone who submitted one of the following suggestions.

*Be gentle with yourself. Learn to say NO and ask for help when you need it. There are occasional days where you must give in to your symptoms, and that's okay.

*Himalayan salt baths are a great way to unwind and relax.

*As broken as you are stay strong. Make peace a priority to protect your physical and emotional state.

*An audiobook is a great way to relax at bedtime. You can drop off to sleep in the middle of a story. Listening to someone else read is soothing and beats lying awake in the dark while everyone else in the house sleeps.

*A full body cushion is inexpensive and an asset for comfort and restless leg syndrome.

*Keep to 1200 calories a day, cut-out processed food, fizzy drinks, confectionery and replace pasteurised milk with almond milk A change of diet can ease depression and stress, which may increase your confidence.

*One cupful of Epsom Salts dissolved in your bath water may ease widespread pain. This is effective just before bedtime.

*Social Services may help with household aids and appliances. There are many useful items available to help you cope better in your home environment. Ring your nearest branch and ask for a home visit to assess you for various household aids which may be available in your area.

*Hire a cleaner if it's within your budget or ask for help. There is no shame in asking anyone to lend a hand or babysit while you catch up on rest.

*Enjoy your good days but don't overdo it. A person with FMS must listen to their body. When you are tired, rest and recuperate.

*You are not obligated to do everything a healthy person does. Stay in bed if you can't get up and never apologise because you're having a bad day. FMS is out of your control. Take it easy on yourself.

*Massage therapy improves pain, anxiety and depression search for a massage therapist who is FMS aware, otherwise you may find yourself in more pain.

*Break big tasks into manageable tasks, adding short rest periods between activities.

*Supplement your diet with flaxseed or fish oil, and ditch caffeine.

*Write detailed notes and use a reminder app on your phone to keep track of important appointments.

*Don't beat yourself up if you need to nap during the day.

*A flannel placed in the freezer for twenty minutes is useful as a cold compress to help neck or localised pain.

*Spend time with people who have a positive outlook and a great sense of humour.

*Watch a funny movie, as laughter can ease pain by releasing brain chemicals that enhance a sense of well-being.

*Focus on things that take your mind off your symptoms You may find this experience rewarding. Experiment with different crafts or classes.

*A massaging foot spa is valuable for people who experience plantar fasciitis or similar foot pain.

*Tips to cope with anxiety attacks. Look around you, find 5 things you can see, 4 things you can touch, 3 things you can hear, 2 things you can smell and 1 thing you can taste. This is grounding. It can help when you are losing control and entering the fight-or-flight mode, of a panic attack.

*Rest or sleep is a necessity while experiencing a severe FMS flare. It is not giving in or giving up, it's self- care.

*Place a plastic chair inside your shower, it's much easier to support personal hygiene.

*Use aids, around the home. I use a kettle tipper, a perching stool and a walking stick. Search for items which may make your life easier.

*Buy a weighted blanket. They are effective while you are dealing with insomnia.

*Supplements such as Vitamin B complex and Magnesium can help with pain and fatigue.

*Join an FMS group to interact with other people who are enduring the same illness. There are several forums and groups on the Internet. You may make friends with fellow sufferers without leaving your home.

*Finally, '**it's okay not to be okay**'.

## Tips to aid Sleep

*Make your bedroom dark and keep the temperature mild.

*A warm shower before sleep is relaxing and will help you unwind.

*Stop caffeine after your evening meal.

*Put your phone out of reach or on silent.

*Aim to get a regular bedtime.

*Try a soothing eye mask. These are valuable to block out light.

*Don't use a tablet, computer, television or phone for at least one hour before bedtime. This can set your thoughts rolling, resulting in an overactive mind.

*If everything else fails and you can't sleep, get up and make yourself a hot drink before trying again.

FMS can present a different scenario every day, and FMS suffers appreciate every hint and tip available to help cope with various coexisting ailments.

# Chapter 8
# **Fibro Facts**

While scrolling through a fibro support group, I noticed a post stating there are several strains of FMS. This is untrue! FMS is one illness which worsens at each distinct stage, it brings other coexisting disorders along, making life more difficult to deal with.

Another contributor stated that the seventh stage of FMS is death. This is not only alarming to those diagnosed, it is also untrue! FMS will not and has not been an attribute to anyone's death. There are no recorded death certificates anywhere, stating FMS is the primary cause of demise.

False information may be alarming to those naïve enough to believe such untruths. More people need educational facts on the disorder.

The following list is factual and may help you understand your condition a little better.

*The two most common debilitating FMS symptoms are widespread pain and CFS.

*Most people diagnosed are middle-aged, although it affects both sexes. Children may also receive a diagnosis.

*Some doctors prefer to use the term growing pains, for any child suffering constant aches.

*80% of people diagnosed are women.

*Eating a rich omega-3 fatty diet may help with joint and muscle stiffness.

*It takes the average patient five years to receive a diagnosis, sometimes it takes longer.

*People with FMS often suffer abnormalities in stage four sleep, which is the stage imperative to restoring and repairing muscles.

*FMS is one of the most common pain conditions worldwide, affecting over two million people in the UK alone.

*You have a debilitating disease, that does not define you as lazy, a liar, a depressive or a crazy person.

*Sleep may not relieve chronic pain, fibro fog or fatigue.

*FMS occurs in all climates, countries and ethnic groups.

*The central nervous system seems to be the underlying factor for FMS patients.

*A person is at higher risk of contracting FMS if they have a rheumatic disease, such as, Osteoarthritis, Rheumatoid Arthritis or Lupus.

*There is no test to detect the disease. It's a matter of rigorous appointments with a variety of GP's and a Rheumatologist.

*Unless you experience the facets of FMS, then it's impossible to understand how a loved one is feeling.

*Self-care is vital to your overall health.

*FMS does not damage muscles, joint and connective tissues.

*FMS is a complex multi system condition, therefore it requires a multi-faceted approach to treatments.

*Rheumatologists consider FMS a musculoskeletal disease because of widespread pain in muscles and joints.

## <u>Just Don't Say It!</u>

While it's often difficult to find the words to provide support and hope for those suffering from FMS, there are some people who speak without thinking and have said:

*You don't look sick!

*Try to get out more!

*Are you imagining it?

*Are you stressed?

*It must be nice not to work!

*Be more positive.

*Go to the doctors, something is depressing you.

*There are many people worse off than you.

*This will pass, you will feel better tomorrow.

*Maybe you have flu.

*It's no good moaning, you must live with it.

*It could be worse.

*If you cannot find the cause of your pain, then it's in your head.

*You need to lose weight!

*You need to do regular exercise!

These statements are upsetting and offensive, when talking to someone who experiences excruciating pain.

Ignore ignorant remarks. Some people may have little understanding on your illness and are unaware how offensive it is for you to hear negative comments.

# Chapter 9
# How Fibromyalgia Affects Your Life

At its worst, FMS is likely to change the way you complete even the smallest task. In this section of the book we will have a look at how different areas of life can require adaptation, and how very easy, daily tasks and ways of life may change for someone diagnosed with FMS.

## **Trouble with Grooming**

As we know that the symptoms of FMS can affect every part of a person's life, it not only has a profound effect on its victims, but can also derail basic manoeuvres and actions which many of us take for granted, destroying one's ability to complete even the most ordinary tasks of daily life.

It might surprise you at how difficult so-called ordinary things have become for sufferers, things that are so basic, that the inability to compete with them can throw a major wrench into their lives.

Considering that FMS affects more women than men, these can be areas that females will often consider as important to their lives, to a greater extent than men will. For instance, personal grooming is such a basic thing for most of us We get up in the morning take a shower, style our hair, and perhaps apply a little make-up, trying to making ourselves presentable to the world.

But, for sufferers of FMS, it is not always as simple as this.

Using the **shower** as an example, the water gets hot which can cause you to become dizzy. The spray of the water, whilst being relaxing and therapeutic for many of us, could be painful to the skin at any temperature for some sufferers. This is thanks to a symptom called **Allodynia**, which means people will experience pain from an unpainful stimulus.

Standing in the shower and using your arms can lead to tired achy muscles. Having a bath instead may eliminate the problems but taking a bath instead of a shower would be much more time consuming and you have the mobility problem of getting in and out of the bath.

Consider styling your own hair. This include manoeuvres such as holding your arms up to brush, blow dry or even straighten or curl your crowning glory, all of which could be tough on the arms. FMS can produce heat sensitivity and styling tools may become a problem. This may also trigger excessive sweating which can undo all your hard work. It may even melt off any make up you have applied. Gone are the days of sitting in a nail or hairdressing salon being pampered, as sitting in one place for any length of time is enough to trigger pain in various parts of your body. Life is tough for us fibro folk.

Wearing clothes is one of the most basic things a human being can do, but this can cause sufferers of FMS a great deal of discomfort. Waistbands, bra straps, the elastic in socks, rough fabrics, tags or labels, or just clothes that are too tight, could all cause pain. Many sufferers will have to tailor or adjust the way they dress to make this less of a problem. Most people with the disorder prefer to wear loose fitting clothing.

Temperature sensitivity can also play a big role selecting clothing too. What can start out as a cosy, comforting sweater on a cold day, can become a baking irritation if we set the heating too high. A cool breeze can make one regret wearing a pair of shorts and a T-shirt or a light cotton shirt.

For those people whom suffer both hot and cold sensitivity, determining what to wear, and enduring the consequences of an incorrect choice, can be disagreeable as you either freeze or overheat, or even alternate between the two.

## The Effects on Social Contact

Sufferers of Fibromyalgia may suffer a certain isolation when their symptoms are chronic, and we saw earlier in this book how FMS blogger, Angela Wise, found herself isolated.

*The symptoms of fatigue and pain you may experience, make healthy levels of social contact with colleagues, family members and friends difficult.

*Talking on the phone can become difficult for sufferers of FMS, but when you have cognitive dysfunction, it may become a problem to even hold the phone for any length of time.

*A few of those diagnosed may even decide it's best they don't drive. It's a personal decision, but one that sufferers will need to consider, as we know that no two days are the same.

## Feeling Overwhelmed.

A common theme with FMS sufferers is feeling overwhelmed. Your life does not stop because you have received an FMS diagnosis, it goes on as before. Children and sometimes elderly parents, require supervision, spouses and partners require attention, household chores mount up as usual, friends and family want to spend time with you and the bills don't stop dropping on the doormat.

Being ill is challenging and may become overwhelming to where you feel lost, isolated, and left without hope. Dealing with FMS while handling life's responsibilities is a daunting task.

Below are a few tips which may help you cope with your emotions and set you on the road to a more positive mind frame, as trying to deal with FMS while handling life's responsibilities is a daunting task.

*If you want to rid yourself of stress, you need to let go of many things in your life.

*Let go of friends and even family unsympathetic to your illness. While this may be difficult, it removes the need to make excuses for your diagnosis and why you feel overwhelmed. Those who don't believe you, don't deserve you.

*If you are feeling overwhelmed, it suggests your mind and body are in a specific state. Try to interrupt that state and go for a short walk if you are able. Pick up the phone and call a sympathetic friend, play some uplifting music or look at photos which recall happy memories.

*Look at the bigger picture. You may realise that many people have been where you are at now and have overcome the same problems you face.

*Start focusing on what you can do instead of the things you cannot control.

*Ask yourself are you a victim or a fibro fighter?

* The journey to feeling better is full of difficulties, it is not linear. When you feel overwhelmed write your feelings in a journal and note what situation, person or event has set this emotion in action.

*Eliminate as much stress from your life as you can. Worrying about situations outside your circle of influence is a waste of your thoughts.

Your body is complex It needs a lot of support which goes beyond diet and nutrition, while diet may play its part, your environment is also important.

If you are feeling overwhelmed, you are not alone and can get out of this cycle, but it requires change and maybe losing a few friends in your inner circle.

# Chapter 10
# **Financial Advice**

While most people diagnosed with FMS will already be aware of their rights to finance, there are those who are unacquainted with the benefits system.

The government introduced several changes to the UK's benefit system. These changes have generated lots of problems. **Universal Credit** received bad publicity as it rolled out across the UK. Claimants have waited five to six weeks for the first payment.

### *Universal Credit

This is a standard allowance which varies depending on a person's age and circumstances. They pay this as a monthly payment, and it includes rents and council tax.

The government suggests the new system is easier to understand and creates incentives for people to work. It has caused chaos across the UK, both council and private landlords have evicted people from their homes and others are using food banks to feed their children. How is this allowed to happen in today's society? Food banks are crying out for donations to keep up the demand from those people waiting on payments. Almost every supermarket asks for customer donations to help their local food banks. We are now in a position where the poor are helping the poor, and many disability organisations worry that some groups of disabled people will get less than they received under the old system.

Perhaps the benefit most people with FMS are reluctant to claim is, Personal Independent Payment (PIPS) This is because of the many horror stories people have shared concerning accessors with little medical training, removing as many people as they can from receiving the benefit. This should not deter you from applying for a benefit you are entitled too.

**\*PIPS** has replaced **Attendance Allowance** and **Mobily Allowance**.

To qualify for this benefit, you must fill in a large detailed form and attend a face-to-face assessment with a medical professional.

There are several horror stories in the media regarding assessors lying and treating people with disrespect. This has led to extreme poverty and even suicide at the unjust scoring system and the assessor's attitude to invisible illness. If FMS were visible, passing the face-to-face assessment would be awarded at first glance.

\*Some assessors profess to know more about your health than you do. If you can walk into the room, they class you able bodied. If you drive you are not eligible, they will find any excuse to disallow this benefit. One ladies skin looked tanned, so they refused her PIPS.

\*To qualify for the **Care Allowance**, you must need help with personal hygiene, dressings, communicating, engaging with other people, preparing or eating food, managing your medication and finances.

\*They award the **Mobility Component** if you have a physical or mental disorder which limits your ability to plan, or follow a journey, or have difficulty moving around.

*They also ask how far you can walk and what aids you use. The assessor will take notice of your mobility as you enter the assessment building and will award points according to his/her judgement.

FMS sufferers do not experience two days the same. You may be immobile for a few days, or you may walk to end of your street another day, with the help of a walking stick. The same applies to care, how can you know from one day to the next, if your body will project widespread pain, stiffness or deliver any other coexisting illness. It's impossible, this is the reason you can't forward plan. Taking this into consideration how do you answer these difficult questions?

Don't put off applying for PIPS, you have a chronic illness which is debilitating. I would advise you to seek help from CAB. They can fill the forms in for you, taking away some of the stress, as the forms are gruelling. There are copious amounts of help from various internet sites to assist you every step of the way.

I asked several FMS people who have attended face-to-face appointments for their advice. I have listed their recommendations for a successful outcome.

*If you cannot attend an examination centre request a home visit.

*Answer the questions explaining how you feel on your worst day.

*Take someone with you to your face-to-face assessment.

*Ask assessors if you may record the interview for your own records as they have been known to bend the truth.

*Write notes and take them with you and if you need to look at them, explain you have fibro fog and didn't wish to leave any information out.

*Take any aids you use to help you walk.

*Don't cover up your illness with make-up the assessor won't see the real you.

*Wear the comfy shoes and clothes you wear every day. Getting dressed up is for parties and you never go out unless it's for hospital or doctor appointments.

*Be honest and tell them your daily struggles.

If your claim is unsuccessful you can ask for a mandatory reconsideration, they will review your claim again and decide if they may change it.

You can appeal the decision through a tribunal which is independent to the **Department of Work and Pensions** (DWP)


In the last four years only 4% of all PIP decisions were overturned at mandatory reconsideration, but at the tribunal stage they overturned most appeals, therefore it's worth your while taking your claim the full way to tribunal.

If, you or your partner claim PIPS, you may receive a disability premium added to your income, if you are in receipt of income-based **Jobseeker's Allowance**, **Housing Benefit** or **Income Support**. If you receive **Universal Credit**, they allow no disability premium.


**Attendance Allowance**:

This award helps you pay for your personal care if you are sixty-five or older and disabled.

**Working Tax Credit**

If you work 16 hours per week, and have received PIPS, you may get an extra amount included in your **Working Tax Credit**.

**ESA:**

This is an allowance paid to people who have a limited ability to work because of sickness or disability. In order to stay on ESA, you must attend a face-to-face medical.

There are many other benefits which some people never think about claiming, yet as a disabled person you are within your right to claim:

*Severe disability payment

*Carers allowance

*A Blue Badge for disability parking

*Disabled persons bus pass

*Car tax discount

*Disabled rail card

*Mobility car. This is only awarded if you receive the enhanced rate on the mobility component of PIPS

If you are in doubt of your right to claim benefits, contact your local CAB office for advice.

# Summary

We know this illness won't kill us, but it will take us on a huge roller coaster ride and present a host of different illnesses. A person with FMs never knows what each day has in store. The worst part of this illness is wondering what tomorrow may bring. If we are lucky, we may experience a few good days a month, but as the disorder progresses the symptoms for most of us appear to worsen.

This illness is destructive it steals our joy. Both our mind and body continuously place roadblocks in our path, so we often surrender to the disorder, and ride out the storm with a dance of pain. We are constantly torn between "I can't allow this disorder to ruin my life", and "I have to listen to my body, rest and recharge".

Good luck on your FMS journey keep fighting and don't allow this destructive illness to define you.

# Part Two
# Fibromyalgia Warriors

# My Wish for You

Comfort on a difficult day,

Smiles when sadness intrudes,

Rainbows to follow the clouds,

Laughter to feel your lips,

Sunsets to warm your heart,

Gentle hugs when spirits sag,

Friendship to brighten your day,

Beauty for your eyes to see,

Confidence for when you are in doubt,

Faith so that you can believe,

Courage to know yourself,

Patience to accept the truth

And love to complete your life.

**Ralf Endo Emerson**

# Fibromyalgia Warriors

The following stories may give you an idea how the human body responds to trauma. I know first-hand how a traumatic experience can throw your body into a chaotic state. When I turned thirty-eight my seven-year old son, Adam, was killed within ten minutes of leaving my home. The person responsible has yet to come forward. My body reacted to the shock by propelling me straight into an early menopause and accelerated the onset of FMS.

Not everyone diagnosed has endured tragedy or trauma. Their illness may come about without cause or reason but most people with the disorder have suffered some form of suffering or distress.

I found writing this part of the book heart wrenching and through this I discovered we are each at different stages of this horrid journey and cope with FMS in our own way.

FMS has overwhelmed some of the contributors. Yet they still found the courage to share their story. They are hoping other sufferers may understand their daily struggles and what they believe triggered their disorder in the first instance.

We may laugh at times or amuse ourselves with unbelievable fibro fog moments, but no one sees what goes on behind closed doors while we are alone. No one knows the traumatic events or tragedies some of us have endured.

It's difficult to dig out dark and depressing events from your memory and to share them with others. This deems everyone who contributed to this section of the book a true *Fibro Warrior*.

I experienced heartache in each of the following stories and shed a few tears, but I gained strength by those contributors who fight this illness with courage and dignity.

# John C

When I noticed a post on a forum asking for people's FMS stories I hesitated.

People assume men to be the stronger sex. This is no disrespect to the ladies who suffer from this illness, I know what you experience. In honesty, my hesitation was, if I recall painful memories, they may drag up a period in my life I have tried so long to forget. After deliberation, I decided my story may help other men to be more open and talk through their own issues on invisible illness and pain.

Apart from the normal scrapes, cuts and bruises I received as a child, I can't recall any major childhood pain. At seventeen, I started a gym. I became addicted to exercise, workouts and healthy eating. At age nineteen, I worked as a doorman at the local nightclub. My life worked well. During the day I went to a gym, at night I worked. Just before my twenty-first birthday an altercation occurred inside the club. My mate Kev walked indoors to see why everyone was fighting. He shouted of me to aid him, as two males and several women were brawling. We separated the bunch and took both males outside, one man winded me by a heavy blow to the stomach. Before I regained my wind, an agonizing pain ripped through my lower stomach. I assumed he had thrown another punch. Both males ran away. I experienced an uncomfortable sensation and hoped I hadn't accidentally urinated. Kev reached for his phone and dialled for an ambulance. I recall thinking who needs an ambulance. I glanced to my feet and saw blood coming from the bottom of my trouser leg; it was then I realised the man had stabbed me. I received surgery to repair the damage from the knife wound and endured a ten-day hospital stay. The surgeon informed me that if the wound been a half an inch to the left, I might have died. The knife man missed a major artery. This was the trigger which set me on a lifetime of pain.

I quit working because of extreme pain which not only affected the site of the wound, it appeared to spread across most of my body. I became weak and listless. The sparkle and love for life I once experienced disappeared. Friends phoned asking if I wanted to go for a gym session or a night out, but I refused making one excuse after another. How could I explain to my mates that pain infiltrated me? They stopped asking and I became a recluse. I refused to visit a doctor to complain of pain. I suppose it's a man thing! This unyielding agony carried on for longer than I expected, it never let up. I received no peace from constant pain and tiredness. I slept every night but woke up feeling exhausted. In the space of six months, I had turned from being a fitness fanatic to a miserable wreck!

Depression crept up on me and swamped my mind. Dark thoughts washed over me at random times. This is when my parents took me to a doctor as I was unable to leave the house on my own. My mother spoke on my behalf as I had become a weepy mess. The help I received from the doctor was amazing. He referred me to a mental health team and a rheumatologist. He diagnosed me there and then with PTSS and FMS.

A glimmer of hope swept over me as I left the surgery with medication and appointments to see two professionals. Maybe a path through the pain and darkness was possible now my illness had a name.

I take medication and the depression is under control. I know my limits and am aware if I go to the gym; I spend the next few days in bed. While my mates are out enjoying their lives, I am in bed by ten o'clock reading. I have learned to take nothing for granted. I go easy on myself and when the pain engulfs me, I talk to people in the same situation. FMS is not only a woman's disease we men also suffer.

# Mandi H

Where do I start? When did FMS invade my body? Both questions are difficult to answer because I honestly have no idea. I have endured a fair few dramas and unpleasant experiences throughout my life. In fact, my life has been one long emotional struggle.

Maybe one or more of the incidents I have experienced triggered FMS and its coexisting illnesses. Was it the car accident I suffered in 2003? A gun held to my head by an alcoholic ex-husband. Or could it be when I performed CPR on my friend's brother? He died of septicaemia. It may even stem from childhood growing pains.

In my younger years, aches and pains were an everyday occurrence which continued into adulthood. My choice of work as a healthcare professional wasn't my best idea, as my immune system was low, and I picked up every bug going.

The ward sister once asked if I had been tested for ME/CFS since my fatigue was noticeable. My job was amazing, but each evening I experienced severe exhaustion after my shift.

In the 2003 car crash I received a severe whiplash. I saw my GP often complaining of widespread pain, he offered no help. It was a frustrating time. In 2010 I got a tattoo on my bottom. In the middle of this procedure, shooting pains travelled up my spine and into my head. The pain became excruciating and the tattooist had to stop. The following day I woke up with a migraine from

78

hell. Since this ordeal my health has deteriorated at an alarming rate. Insomnia prevents me from sleeping, fibro fog affects my memory, I experience widespread pain daily and migraines continue to plague me. I attempted a return to work but found it impossible. They released me from my contract on the grounds of ill health.

I asked my GP if my symptoms were comparable to FMS His abrupt response took me by surprise. He said, "No, fibromyalgia doesn't exist. It is a name given to people when a doctor has no diagnosis for his patient". He sent me for a celiac disease test and referred me to an immunologist. I endured various investigations before they diagnosed me with FMS and M.E. My own diagnosis was correct.

My husband became redundant and is now my primary carer. I rely on his help every day in order to function.

Loose pyjamas are my best friend as most fabric irritates my sensitive skin. We installed a wet room as using a bath became impossible. I cannot cook, clean or do tasks normal people complete every day. Sleep is not refreshing and restorative. I may sleep during the day or through the night and still wake exhausted. I use a walker or a wheelchair. This depends if I am well enough for an outing and the severity of my pain.

This forbidding illness has steered me to the depths of hell. I attempted suicide as this illness left me a former shadow of myself. Had it not been for my husband's quick thinking, I may not have survived. FMS has taken over my life. Day by day, it continues to destroy what little independence I have. It is cruel and unyielding, yet I still rise each day hoping the day brings happiness.

My story may sound despondent and gloomy, but I want people to know how I am attempting to overcome adversity. I have experienced anger, disbelief and a lack of self-worth, but I realise that life is a gift, and we should live it the best way we can with whatever illness we may endure. Now that you know my life story, I will leave it in the past and look forward to a brighter tomorrow.

# Denise H

My childhood was difficult. I tuck the memories of abuse and pain to the back of my mind. To bring them forward is as painful as the illness which batters my body. I have heard people say trauma may be the trigger for FMS. My life has been one long traumatic event. They suggested I experienced growing pains as a child, but I know my pain came from a different source. FMS was unheard of in my younger years. Today it's a different story. People of all ages are diagnosed even children.

As I got older, I found myself in one disastrous relationship after another. I suffered a different form of abuse with each destructive partner I chose. They each had demons and I picked up the pieces from internet sex addiction, alcohol abuse and gambling, which resulted in severe financial difficulties. My stress levels went through the roof and widespread pain became a daily occurrence.

In 2010 the doctors diagnosed rheumatoid arthritis and two years later they detected FMS. My GP is excellent I can't find fault in the treatment I receive. The rheumatology department is not so helpful. I believe they lack the funds to run an efficient unit. I am on an excellent medication regime. Certain medications are unsuitable because of a drug sensitivity but I cope by eliminating those which cause problems.

My positive outlook to life and a high pain threshold, places me in a better situation than those fibro friends who find this appalling disease difficult to handle. I hold a full-time work position as an Adult Protection Social Worker. The work is stressful, but my employers are superb. They make reasonable adjustments with equipment. They also allow me to work from home if I can't attend. I try to condense my hours into four days which allows me a full day at home to recover.

Several other conditions have caused problems. A gallbladder removal and pressure on my brain, caused huge FMS flares. I keep my life busy; this takes my mind away from my illnesses, but FMS lets me know when to stop and recharge. Then I start over again. It's a never-ending cycle. I have smiled behind silent tears, cried behind closed doors and I fight hard to win this battle. It won't beat me.

I don't look back to the past, it's pointless and painful. My aim is to move forward as I have two stunning daughters and three adorable grandchildren who keep me on my toes. I pray they do not inherit FMS or suffer the same fate as myself. My advice to others with an invisible illness is; "Life is tough, but so are you. Stay strong and take each day as it's comes."

# Tanya B

I can't remember a time I haven't experienced pain. As a small child I suffered abuse and neglect. My early memories weren't pleasant. I didn't have the best start to life. My alcoholic stepfather constantly shouted and displayed violent behaviour towards me. I became withdrawn. I often experienced pain at a young age, but never mentioned it for fear of more abuse. In adolescence I avoided being in the family home as much as possible. I often stayed at an aunt's house to evade the sadistic behaviour. A friend's mother observed how I winced when I moved and asked me if I was ill. I explained I suffered with constant widespread pain. She took me to my family doctor who prescribed codeine phosphate. The pains didn't vanish, but the codeine helped me experience normality. I left home and went to live with my aunt. Several years later, I took more tablets than the doctor prescribed, and I became codeine dependant. Without my daily fix I experienced problems. Once my aunt noticed my medications were not lasting, she took me back to the doctors for further advice. I explained how pain had took over my life, but the doctor shook his head and disagreed. He sent me to a detox group. I became so frustrated. No one listened. I experienced abnormal pain and they took my medication away. They dismissed me as an unruly teen addicted to prescription medication. I felt alone and lost.

I met my partner Joe and together we made a nice home. Joe accompanied me to the doctors and tried to explain my symptoms. The doctor refused to prescribe pain relief because of the earlier addiction. He refused to refer me to a pain clinic and suggested I had a depressive nature. I experienced depression, but it stemmed back to childhood memories.

One morning I woke up confused I didn't realise which day of the week it was, and I couldn't move my limbs. Joe assumed I was having a stroke. He called an ambulance and I was taken to hospital. I endured various tests, and they referred me to a psychiatric councillor and a rheumatologist. I received answers. My pain wasn't imagined, it was real! They told me the trauma of my childhood had caused JFMS. Junior Fibromyalgia Syndrome, which had worsened over the years. After several visits to a psychologist and a rheumatologist, I started a treatment plan. Someone believed me, I was ecstatic.

My life is still not pain free although over the counter medication helps. I suffer with constant fatigue and widespread pain along with acute fibro fog. I put my mobile phone in the freezer and the television remote in the microwave. It's funny trying to find things. Joe's support is unreal. I dread to think how my life may have turned out had I not met him.

I spend four days a week in bed because of widespread pain. Joe brings me hot water bottles to place on sore areas and massages my limbs which helps. I may get dressed once a week, but I spend my days in pyjamas. Using the shower is exhausting but I go in every other day. Joe often dries me as it depletes my energy. I only fight this illness because of the kindness shown by my partner and his family. I avoid my immediate family since stress exaggerates my symptoms.

No doctor will prescribe pain medication because of addiction issues. I am bitter that no one detected my illness when I was younger, then maybe my life could have been happier. A life with FMS is gruelling but I am slowly learning how to cope.

# Charlotte W

My first child was double breech. I experienced a natural birth and the pain was excruciating. From that day onward I suffered horrific pain in my hips which I associated to the traumatic delivery. My next birth was as traumatic. I opt for a spinal tap, but the doctors experienced a problem inserting the epidural and hit my spine three times with the needle. This is the trigger which began my journey with FMS.

Not long after the first birth I dislocated my ankle and the agony from my both my hip and foot became unbearable. The pain crept to various parts of my body and my coping mechanisms were zero. Every day became a living hell. I visited the doctor regularly complaining of widespread pain. Convincing him my pain was real became a chore. Why people assumed I imagined illness is beyond me. After several visits getting nowhere, I stood firm and told the doctor that something was wrong. He sent me to a specialist who diagnosed me with FMS and scoliosis. I experienced depression and anxiety, my days were pain filled and dark. No one understood how ill and lethargic I had become.

Chronic fatigue became a regular symptom often sending me to bed. The medication prescribed makes me drowsy and sleepy but it's not a refreshing sleep. I always appear worn out and frazzled.

I am blessed with a good partner he supports and looks after me. I should be grateful, but I find myself wishing my life away. Wishing to run around with my ten-year-old daughter, wishing to go back to my job of hairdressing, wishing the pain away and wishing my life was normal. I force myself to get dressed only to lie on the sofa. Sunday is different; I stop in pyjamas throughout the day. What a life! The pain has become widespread and every day I appear to develop a new symptom. My eyesight is atrocious and it's getting worse. I can't say I have a particular coping mechanism. I turn to my medications and suffer the side effects. My ten-year-old daughter cares for me. We go to bed at the same time. It's sad for her to have a disabled mum, but she takes it in her stride and helps as much as she can.

FMS has ruined my life. Bit by bit this illness has attacked my body. Every part of me has experienced the force of FMS. I wish to go back to work and offer financial support for my family but it's impossible. Fibro Fog is another blight on my life, my memory is shocking. I have stood in a shop doorway and then forgot why I went. When I ponder on my life, the daily pain and chronic fatigue, I am not sorry for myself, it's my child who grabs my pity. I am sorry for the life I am unable to offer her.

My fears for the future rests with her as she often complains of joint pain. FMS runs in my family. My sister received a diagnosis and my mum is showing symptoms. My doctor informed me this may be an inherited condition. At present I await a referral back to my specialist.

# Mary U

I suppose everyone experiences trauma sometime or another. Throughout the years I have had my share of harrowing events. I can only describe the younger years of my life as swimming in stormy waters against the tide.

By the time I reached seventeen I had married and given birth to a baby girl. I set up home and began the role of wife and mother. Throughout these early years we experienced problems. A few cracks appeared in our marriage. How we endured the challenges thrown our way I don't know, but we survived to celebrate our golden wedding anniversary this year.

I gave birth to three children and each of them weighed over 10lb When I delivered my second child, he was huge and double breech. A doctor performed an episiotomy and used forceps to aid the delivery. The birth traumatised me from start to finish. I assumed this ordeal contributed to the early onset of this disorder. As the years passed, I endured several operations to correct a bladder issue. In one medical procedure a negligent surgeon left part of a finger cot inside my body while I was being stitched. He knew of this issue but never informed me; he expected the finger cot to pass via my vagina when the stitches dissolved. It did not! They later discovered, this foreign body had migrated through the bladder wall and had formed a calculus mass. So, through medical negligence, I ended up with an urostomy bag and the full onset of FMS.

I am at the last stage where I accept this illness and its coexisting problems. My life is a car crash and I am fighting hard to live amid the wreckage. My quality of life is poor, as is my mobility and I live with perpetual pain. I watch television in bed or rest on a reclining chair doing puzzles. I do not live a productive or exciting life. My energy levels are zero, they are non-existent. I can't cook, clean or do the smallest of tasks without suffering the consequences as everything exhausts me. Resting is my way of getting through every single day. How I grieve for the old version of me, for losing my mobility, for losing cognition and losing my identity. This illness has changed me beyond recognition.

My legs struggle to keep me upright as my leg muscles have wasted. My last pain free day has faded from my memory. Most people are judgemental and call me lazy. I am not lazy. My body is weary and exhausted from trying to restore itself. I cope with my other morbidities to the best of my ability, but this illness is unyielding.

The worst part of my illness is the recurring judgement from those who don't care enough to research FMS or observe my daily widespread pain. They say my illness is invisible, yet I see it each time I glimpse at my reflection.

# Paula H

They say a virus, or a traumatic event can trigger FMS. I've experienced more traumas than most. My life has been one of tragedy and distress. In fact, I don't know where to begin. I suppose my life was normal until the age of twenty-three. After receiving fertility treatment, I lost two babies. My third pregnancy resulted in the baby being born at twenty weeks gestation. She weighed only 2lb 6oz.

They diagnosed me with FMS when I was twenty-six years old. The doctors thought the stress of losing my babies and the difficult birth began my journey with a lifelong illness.

I often wonder why me? I found my mother dead one Thursday, the following day somebody murdered my brother. How much can one woman endure? I became a victim of PTSS I was no pleasure to be around. Depression engulfed my whole being. It became a dark period in my life. I lost my husband because he didn't consider me fun. The spark that held our marriage together went out. This took my spark for life away.

I tried to cope the best way possible and met up with an old school friend. We developed a connection and fell in love. I found him dead from a heart attack four months into the relationship. How unjust! Life kept dealing me tragedy after tragedy. Why me? What have I done to deserve these merciless life experiences?

Depression strikes around 90% of the time. I live a lonely and sad life and can't see any prospects of a meaningful existence ahead of me. They've prescribed me antidepressants, but they can't heal my past or improve my future, so the pain and depression cycles continue.

I always cancel plans as I can't predict from one day to the next how my illness will affect me. I can't go out with friends, since I suffer from a lack of self-confidence, tiredness and anxiety. What infuriates me is that no one can imagine my pain. Unless you have FMS, you could never understand the severity of this debilitating illness. I always have flu symptoms minus the runny nose and other side effects of flu. It's the constant nagging ache of muscles tendons and ligaments that causes me widespread pain. My body is under attack! On a scale of 1-10 my pain levels are around 7 on a good day. The pain goes way off the chart when a fibro flare knocks me sideways. When this occurs every part of my body hurts even my skin hurts to touch. What a life!

I can't tolerate loud noises or listen to someone talking while the television is playing. It's just too much for me to handle. I lost my PIPS three year ago and I refused to appeal. The thought of facing a tribunal or endless form filling sends me spiralling into an anxiety attack so I receive nothing. I think the government's policy on PIPS is shocking. My health is chronic, but I am denied benefits. Dealing with professional people is a huge problem, I find talking to strangers difficult; I freeze, and the words won't flow. That scenario could propel me straight into a panic attack and I can't allow for that to happen.

I have several pyjama days per week and prefer not to get dressed, but I make the effort as I take my grandchild to school on a morning. It's just out of my back gate which makes it easier. My weekends are pyjama days. I can't see the point in getting dressed and I find pyjamas are gentler against my skin which hurts to the touch. Along with FMS, I have Graves' disease, Arthritis, COPD, IBS and the list continues to grow.

My life is tough but other people's lives are tougher. That doesn't mean I count my blessings as my life has been harrowing and difficult. One thing I am sure of is, somewhere deep inside of this frail body there dwells a fighting spirit which won't give in or give up the fight. Whatever else is in store for me I will survive as surviving is the only way I know how to live.

# Marion. H

I was a normal happy child but at age fourteen I experienced something no child should endure, sexual abuse This spiralled my lifelong journey with depression. I tried to tuck the memory of this ordeal to the back of my mind, but it often comes to the fore and haunts me. This is the trigger which opened the doorway to poor health.

People often commented that I was the outgoing friend, but they did not see what lay behind my smile. My life has seen its share of good and bad times. The bad often outweighed the good. After a failed marriage I picked myself up and started again. Once my children lived independent lives, I began a new job. It was enjoyable and my colleagues became friends, but bouts of unspeakable pain and depression washed over me and it became uncontrollable regardless of which medication I took.

I met a nice gentleman and we became a couple. Over a six-month period, he displayed narcissistic behaviour. I escaped this destructive relationship and picked up the pieces of my shattered life, but every day became a struggle. Stress produced panic attacks and I developed a lack of self-worth. Words could not describe the widespread pain which battered my body every day. There was no other alternative but to resign from my job as I was chronically fatigued, worn out and, suffered unyielding low moods. It was one of the lowest periods of my life. In fact, my life fell apart.

My FMS diagnosis took a long time. If only they had looked deeper into my pain fuelled life, I may have received the help I needed quicker. I've always sustained what life has thrown at me, but I must now admit defeat. Suicide has crossed my mind, but I couldn't see my family suffer the consequences, so I remind myself that amid the pain, frustration and fog, I will push forward and continue living this hell!

The fibro fog is hard to cope with. It takes over my mind and I lack the concentration needed to complete any basic tasks. How my life has changed! The Marion who hid behind her smile has vanished. My smiles are rare these days. My bed days are around three at present and climbing. FMS attacks every part of my body and no magic pills are available to fix me. Insomnia is the bane of my life. I spend most days in bed, but it doesn't mean I get restorative sleep. It's the reverse. Sleep doesn't come often and when it does it's not a deep restful sleep.

My friends and family know that if I don't answer the phone or I cancel plans at the last moment; it's not because I don't care, it's because I need to take care of myself. I am bitter at the lack of support from my doctor. I still fight to get believed. My pain is real and not imagined. I am not a crazy depressed hypochondriac. I live with pain daily. We need more sympathetic doctors to understand the needs of people with FMS and we deserve support.

# Christina C

They say God only gives us what we can endure. I am at my limit and can take no more, for if I experience further adversity, I will lose my sanity.

I am twenty-nine years old and I can't recall a period in my life where pain hasn't affected me. The doctors suggest my FMS first began from the age of nine. I believe I was younger than this. A traumatic event can trigger FMS, but how far back can your memories take you? Do injurious things happen while we are young and get tucked to the back of our minds?

When I turned thirteen, I discovered sexual abuse had taken place when I was two years old. I am left wondering if this ordeal projected physical pain during my younger years.

Throughout my childhood I complained of aches pains, sore joints and fatigue. I could not tolerate any weight on my legs. I experienced pin and needles, blurred vision, sleeping problems and loss of movement in my limbs. My hospital visits were too many to count. A simple bug wiped me out for six weeks. My diagnosis was growing pains. Why do doctors insist on this nonsensical diagnosis?

At age seventeen I gave birth to my first child, he was premature. The following three births were traumatic. My body gave up after the deliveries and on two occasions my life was at risk.

When I reached twenty-three my body turned against me. I endured a spate of falls which resulted in hospital visits for sprains, tendon and ligament damage. It was difficult to understand why this was happening to me. It felt so wrong. Fatigue became the bane of my life. It left me unable to complete a simple task and I needed help. Widespread pain along with depression overwhelmed me and became a daily part of my existence.

I was in a wheelchair with four children and a home to attend. The doctor referred me for scans, bloods and an MRI. I then received a diagnosis of osteoarthritis and FMS, along with anxiety and Bipolar. I understand why I experience mental health issues as trauma has become a way of life from me.

I thought things couldn't get any worse, but it did! My four children each developed serious health issues. The oldest son developed ADHD, my ten-year-old daughter has received a diagnosis of JFS, (Juvenile Fibromyalgia Syndrome) My third son suffers with Tourette's and Autism and my youngest child has ADHD and Autism. Each day brings a new problem into our household.

To add further misery to my blighted life, I live in a three-storey town house and they situated the bathroom on the top floor. The stairs are too narrow to fit a stair lift, so life is a struggle. I am trying to find a home which better suits our needs. I hope this happens soon.

You may wonder how I cope. I often ask myself the same question. My nan and mum cannot offer much support as they each have FMS This relentless illness has inflicted havoc on our family. It attacks each generation. FMS is the primary cause of my pain, but I won't allow the pain to destroy my life. The odds are against me, but I don't intend to give up. I will fight this illness every day and give my children the attention they need.

# Dianne C

My journey started as a small child. I have endured pain for as long as I can remember. A doctor diagnosed me with growing pains and hypermobility at a young age. Why professionals diagnose growing pains in children is beyond me. Is there such a thing? I suffered pain no child should endure, and this was not because of a growth spurt. Nothing eased the constant nagging ache. This continued throughout my childhood and when puberty set in at a young age the pain intensified.

Chronic fatigue hit me hard when I turned twenty. My doctor diagnosed anxiety and depression. The medication had side effects which made me drowsy; this worsened my abnormal fatigue. I knew my own body, and something was not right.

Working as a carer both in a care home and for a private client was a demanding job. I used to come in and collapse on the couch. My limbs were heavy and aching. My life revolved around work and pain relief. Sometimes I managed an occasional night out with friends.

My body turned against me and each day brought a new battle to fight. I couldn't go on any longer. Work suffered because of my failing health. I resigned from my job to take care of myself. After many visits to doctors and specialists they informed me I had FMS. It came as no surprise. Both my sister and nephew suffer the same illness. I am still of the opinion my doctor doesn't understand the full scale or the impact this illness throws my way. I was forty-two when they diagnosed me. My life may have been easier if the doctors had listened instead of prescribing the wrong medication.

I miss the old me, even with the level of pain I experienced. My life was manageable, and I often enjoyed a laugh with colleagues and friends. I even enjoyed the odd cuppa at friends' home. How different my life is now! The days I look well are rare and less frequent.

Other people's attitudes annoy me, just because I smile does not mean I am pain free. You may see me around the village or in the shops, but that doesn't mean my pain has vanished. When I say, "I am fine" I am not but I can't keep moaning to people. This disorder is invisible, but I am not! I am a caring human being that has a debilitating illness, I live with it every day and I can never be sure what part of my body it will attack next.

This cruel illness has changed me. I am no longer the person I used to be. My independence has vanished. My head is above water but inside I am drowning. Last year they diagnosed me with a stroke, yet the MRI came back normal. The doctor told me I had suffered a serious flare. What more can this illness throw at me? I hurt in places unimaginable, at a level beyond your comprehension but don't offer me any sympathy. I don't want it. Show me you understand. I am fifty-six years old now and I don't think my future will get better. Sometimes I fear for what lies ahead. I survive a high level of pain, emotional trauma, guilt, cognitive dysfunction and sleep deprivation along with relentless fatigue. My quality of life is poor, and it won't get any better. It's destroying me from the inside out. FMS is part of my life, but it does not define me. My strength and courage do. I will battle whatever this illness throws my way with dignity.

# Leighann J

Is our fate predetermined or did I draw the short straw for continuous traumatic events? I guess I will never know. I can say with certainty from the age of fifteen, I have endured unbearable ordeals, as vivid today as they were when each occurred. My journey began while I attended school on an army base in Germany. While lying on the top bunk in our dormitory, a flash of light followed by a huge explosion lit up the room. The windows shattered and covered me with glass. The IRA had planted a car bomb near our sleeping quarters. I became withdrawn and fatigued, often nodding off in lessons. I suffered bouts of widespread pain which the doctor diagnosed as depression. He prescribed me various medications to aid sleep and help with anxiety. Could this be the trigger which caused FMS to rip through my body? Or maybe, it was the move to Northern Ireland with a narcissistic husband?

We had two children together and my husband controlled every part of our lives. I became chronically fatigued and fell asleep without having his meal ready. It was the ultimate sin in his eyes. He informed me he was sending me home with a placard around my neck stating, *"RETURNED AND REJECTED"*. This egotistical man made my life hell. He refused to let me take the children back home to England, so my only escape from a pain and horror filled life was death. I overdosed but failed. His cruelty continued by poisoning the children's minds against me. It took my sanity which secured me a place in a psychiatric unit because of my continuous attempts at death. I left

Northern Ireland defeated, depressed, in pain and heart broken. He stole years of my life and my two children.

I continued to experience chronic widespread pain, depression and fatigue but I met a sweet gentleman who I thought kind. I was so wrong! He beat my body black and blue and broke my wrists. To escape another terrible relationship, I ran away while he was sleeping. I got a train back to my mothers with one bag of clothing. Another trigger?

I met someone else, married and had a further three children. The marriage became unstable, he often walked out for no reason. During this time, he had three affairs. Each time it happened my body produced more pain. He called me lazy and a hypochondriac. Eighteen years later I found the strength to kick him out of the marital home. He continued to make my life hell for a further two years and my body projected further pain, fatigue and other morbidities. My life became a continuous battle for survival.

One doctor suggested my symptoms were comparable to FMS and sent me for further testing. I received a diagnosis in March 2013. It was a huge relief knowing I was not lazy or a hypochondriac as other suggested. My illness was real.

I suffer from severe fatigue, and my pain is never below 7 on a pain scale rating. My life as a single parent is difficult. I can't interact with my children as other parents do. There are days when depression strikes. I have no control over this.

My daughter helps me with my hygiene needs. Without her I could not shower, she is my rock. Cooking is impossible. I microwave most meals and cannot execute any household chores, put clothes in the washing machine or cook.

Every task is exhausting. I loved taking my dogs for a walk but it's an impossible feat. At present I am waiting for two knee replacements. I hope this helps with my mobility. I am aware the years ahead of me are pain filled as FMS is incurable. A stair lift is a necessary aid. It enables me a small bit of freedom as I have been a prisoner trapped in my bedroom. There are various other aids to help me around the house, but my daughter is my lifeline to normality. How sad my life has come to this, and how sad that my daughter has so much responsibility on her young shoulders.

FMS brought a storm into my life when I turned fifteen, but life has shown me; I am a survivor of storms. I am a **_Fibro Warrior_**.

# Erica

I can't remember childhood pain but in my teenage years, I suffered with an unnatural tiredness. I had zero energy and couldn't run around as others my age did.

At eighteen I became pregnant and I married at twenty. By the time I was twenty-three another two children had arrived. It was difficult attending three little ones along with a demanding husband. My marriage was harrowing, and it didn't last long. I divorced and brought the children up on my own. I was twenty-four when painful swollen fingers plagued me. It was around this time depression struck and the doctor prescribed me medication; it is still on my repeat prescription list today along with a multitude of others.

I only received an FMS diagnosis three years ago, but I know I have had this illness longer than they suggest. I visit my doctor so often he sighs when he sees my name; although he listens and has organised scans and further tests.

My life is a struggle. Every day is a different challenge. There are days I lock the doors and hide away as I don't want to engage in chat with anyone. Other days I motivate myself to complete basic hygiene tasks, such as getting washed or brushing my hair. I only dress if I need to see someone or get somewhere, as it's a hassle getting ready for any outing. Most people don't realise how exhausting simple tasks can be. Bras are a nightmare for me as are socks. It's the simple things normal people take for granted that I find so frustrating. I take a nap every afternoon.

If I am extra fatigued, I will lie on the couch most of the day. This does not define me as lazy; I am not feigning illness I have a lifelong disorder. Each day I try my best to cope with whatever malady is upon me. FMS was the reason I resigned from work, the pain was too much to cope with and my time keeping was rubbish.

Arthritis affects most of my joints along with crippling pain in my legs and feet. This pain keeps me awake at night. I receive steroid injections into the bursa on both hips. What a life! Oh, I forgot to mention the headaches that pound my head until the pain is unbearable, and no one can tell me why they occur? The neurologist informed me migraines were not to blame, so I plod on and take what medication I am prescribed. Life is not a bed of roses. It's far from easy. I don't ponder on the future. I take each day as it comes and hope tomorrow may be brighter.

FMS is a journey I never planned or asked for, but I fight this illness every day of my life. I do not believe they will find a cure in my lifetime. I hope future sufferers may not have to endure the same fate. More people need education about this invisible illness.

# Maria P

I experienced a normal loving family life as a child and can recall lots of happy memories My problems began when I developed a relationship which turned out to be violent and abusive. This lasted for twelve years. When I escaped and started a new life, I experienced dull aches and pains but thought this was general fatigue. When the pain became a real problem, I visited my doctor who diagnosed me with a B12 deficiency along with a thyroid disorder.

My doctor gave me B12 injections. He assumed the root cause of every illness was a lack of this vitamin. He appeared to show little interest in me, and I convinced myself he labelled me a hypochondriac. My symptoms were real; I experienced widespread pain along with memory loss and abnormal tiredness. My imagination didn't invent these symptoms. No one has ever offered me an explanation to why my body produces profound pain. I find this neglectful.

At the time of my diagnosis, I hadn't heard of FMS.I am bitter towards my doctors for their lack of care and their failure to give me basic facts about this illness.

FMS fuels most days with pain, some days are mild others are crucifying. I drag myself out of bed to go to work. Other days I phone in sick. My life revolves around pain, fatigue, memory loss and trying to please everyone. There are people who don't understand my daily struggles. I have lost countless friends since I am unreliable to attend any events they arrange. Each day is different as this disorder produces a multitude of symptoms.

I need to change doctors maybe one who can sympathise and understands my problems. Trying to get this illness under control myself without support is impossible. I am limited to what I can and cannot do. When I try to join in a social night or event, I end up in bed for two days with severe and unnatural pain, imagining I am dying a slow painful death. No one understands my plight and I am sure most people think I exaggerate my symptoms and often sigh when I mention my struggles. I don't fake being sick, I fake being well.

If I had had more knowledge on this disorder in my youth and was told trauma may cause illness, my life may be different today. It is unfortunate we can't know which individuals make unsuitable partners until it's too late. I didn't ask for FMS, but it attacked my body and I must live with it for the rest of my life. This cruel illness scares me, and I wonder how I will cope as I get older. It's a horrible disease and my heart aches for those who suffer day in and day out.

I am still without medication. I am trying hard to get help. The doctors appear to show little interest and my depression worsens. The only medication I receive are antidepressants, but the side effects are extreme. FMS has taught me that life is tough for people with invisible illnesses. I will cope with the negative sides of this disorder as I have little choice in the matter. My only wish is those around me including the doctors, were more understanding.

# Jane S

I am lying on my bed in tears; I cry often. This illness is unrelenting, and I am unsure how much more I can endure. I cry bitter tears, but I am not depressed; I am lonely, sad, lost and afraid of the future. Most of my tears are for a broken body which refuses to heal.

I hate my bedroom it is my jail. I glance around the room and see smart furniture, velvet bedding, matching curtains and a television on an ornate stand. Everything is gleaming but it's a prison cell and I am serving a life sentence. My illness is invisible but when I look in the mirror hanging on the cell wall, I notice heavy dark circles around my eyes. My skin is pallid and the spark for life that once bounced back at me in a reflection has vanished. I glance back in the mirror and speak out loud. "Fibromyalgia, I see you and I suffer your cruelty."

This illness attacks when I least expect it. It has many facets. I am defeated, FMS has won. I haven't had the best of lives but at least I was free and not trapped inside a shattered body. My tears are not for the abuse and devastation I have suffered during my life, they are for the lost years that FMS has stolen.

I no longer experience the joy and excitement of packing for a holiday or preparing for a road trip to visit family. I miss the sun on my joints, dancing, nights out with friends and family and I miss the old me. The happy, energetic and talkative old Jane has vanished and a newer version of me, with no zest for life has occupied my body.

My words may sound despondent, but they are from my heart. I know FMS won't shorten my life but it sure as hell causes me copious amounts of excruciating pain.

I may manage my illness better if the pain stayed in one part of my body, but it's widespread and I can't pinpoint which area hurts the most. My days revolve around medication, natural therapy, heated wheat bags and television. Tomorrow is a new day, but it holds no joy for me, as I wonder what this insistent disorder has planned.

I will endure FMS as I have no choice, but how nice it must be to be normal once again. I suppose depression has taken hold of me as it's difficult to see a brighter road ahead.

Telling my story has had a therapeutic effect. It's made me realize I need professional help to conquer this depression. I intend to speak to my GP and explain my sadness.

Maybe there's a light at the end of the tunnel I hope so, and perhaps with time the old Jane may return.

# Mary S

I experienced growing pains around the age of ten. While growing up I was an anxious child, maybe this resulted from the beatings I received which may be a contributing cause to my illness. I cannot say this caused my body to project profound pain. It is only my theory.

I suffered with extreme pain for years before my diagnosis in 2010. I informed my doctor of the struggles I faced. He never mentioned FMS, he dismissed my illness as depression. I told him I was struggling to lift my arms. I couldn't even put washing on a line. He laughed and said, "It's the same for everyone". I didn't go back as he intimidated me, and I felt silly for mentioning it. I knew my symptoms were real and not imagined. You can't imagine pain. It exists, it's real! When I finally received an FMS diagnosis years later my doctor apologised for not recognising the symptoms earlier, and for his failure in providing the correct pain relief.

These days I muddle along the best I can. My head wants to do things, but my body can't follow. Constant tiredness and pain ruin my quality of life. I am shattered each morning as pain wakes me up every few hours which prevents restorative sleep.

The pain originates in various areas of my body. I struggle to get out of bed or walk, so if I need the toilet during the night I shuffle along the landing. My bed days are around two to three times a week.

I struggle to get up each morning to attend to my cats and dog. This not only wears me out, but it saddens me. There are days I stay in pyjamas as getting dressed is exhausting. Hospitals are the only places I visit at present. I take twelve different medications, but four of them are for Atrial Fibrillation and COPD. The medication numbs the pain but the longer I take it the less effective it works. It makes me dizzy and nauseous, tired and listless. Weight gain is another side effect, not through overeating as my appetite is poor. I eat to live, not to enjoy. FMS has cost me my confidence and a zero-social life. I lost friends, they just drifted away.

My life took a downward spiral when I resigned from my job due to deteriorating health issues.

They say every cloud has a silver lining, mine comes in the form of my three daughters. They each lead constructive lives of their own yet still find time to help me out in any way they can.

The worst part of my illness is, not being able to have my grandchildren sleepover as they once did. I can't care for the younger ones any longer. My older grandchildren are a great comfort and often help me with various jobs. They take me out in a wheelchair but when I return home, it's straight to bed to recover. I smile because it's expected of me but at times I long to be alone. I am sure people get fed up of me moaning. My future is not good or bright. When I look to the forthcoming days and months ahead, I envisage pain, medication and doctor's appointments. FMS has taken over my body and is sucking the life from me. My future is not bright, it's painful.

People who have never experienced chronic pain can't understand the exhaustion and fatigue I experience or the problems this illness throws at me. FMS has changed my life; it has changed me as a person. My days are a roller coaster ride, one day I am up the next I am down, and the ride never ends, but I refuse to let this illness beat me. I make the most of good days which don't occur often, but they are still worth living.

# Tracey C

Have I ever sensed normality? To be honest, I don't think I have! I remember pain ripping through my joints when I was just four years old. It's an alarming place to be when your health declines especially when your life is just beginning.

I lived a normal life, but it always included widespread pain. My mother became worried and carted me off to a doctor who diagnosed growing pains and hypermobility. I became excluded from physical exercise at school. No one believed how much pain I endured as a child. My mother paid for a doctor's note often, which sufficed the teachers and excused me from taking part in any strenuous games. I longed to be normal and join in the fun with my school friends. They excluded me from various activities, and I turned out to be a lonely child.

When I turned fifteen my doctor diagnosed lumbago. I thought he was insane for suggesting this but looking back he had no other explanation as to why my body produced profound pain every single day.

When I turned twenty my dad died, he was only forty-four years old. Stress swallowed me whole then spit me out; not only had I lost my father I had to arrange his funeral. My anxiety levels were through the roof and I experienced chronic fatigue. This was severe and caused more problems. After visiting my doctor yet again, he listened and sent me for tests. I can never forget the doctor's words when he presented me with a diagnosis. He said, "Tracey, you have FMS now you can get on with your life.". That's it! No words of advice and no sympathetic ear. I cried with frustration. I had a diagnosis, but no treatment. This was one period in my life where I experienced a deep sense of despair.

I met and married my wonderful husband. We started a family immediately. After the birth of my first son Daniel, we were happy, but my health deteriorated even further. I became exhausted and in pain, but life had to go on. I had a husband, home and a child who required care.

Reflecting on my past I don't have a clue how I managed the exertion. Every day became more of a struggle. Hope of a better tomorrow was the fuel that kept me going.

I often ponder on this period in my life and wonder how the hell I coped. I fell pregnant a second time but miscarried. More stress! My third pregnancy pushed my anxiety levels through the roof. I bled at twenty weeks and my second son was born ten weeks early. One trauma after another plagued me. I filled my days by looking after the boys, trying to keep on top of housework and cope with widespread pain.

My life has not been easy and my health continues to deteriorate, but I plod on each day hoping tomorrow may be better.

My pain levels are so severe I take my prescribed morphine more often than I should, sometimes up to 300ml in a two-week period. I am often waiting for my next prescription before it's due. The medications I receive helps, but it's unjust how my life revolves around an assortment of pain relief to exist. The housework is mounting up in my home which depresses me. Any small task spirals my body to unimaginable pain. I am not a lazy person but it's impossible to achieve the smallest of tasks although I try my best.

My heart aches for my husband. I went through early menopause when I was thirty-two. My libido vanished. He tells me not to worry as sex is the last thing on his mind. He still loves me even with my illness. He is one of a kind.

I make the most of each day. I accept my health will not improve; it will get worse as this illness claws its way through my body inch by inch. Both my boys are grown up now and live constructive lives of their own. My grandchildren are adorable, and I wish to see them grow up and flourish. I intend to fight this illness in any way I can.

# Carol E

I suffered a normal home life as a child until my eighth birthday. I can never forget this day. My father's friend raped me. When I look back on my childhood the worst part of the attack besides the pain was being branded a liar. My mother either didn't want to believe it was true or thought I was attention seeking. A child does not question adults so I assumed it must have been my fault. I lived with the attack on my mind throughout my younger years. I still shudder when I recall that dreadful day.

I married twice. Both relationships failed and I set up home for the third time with my three children. Stacey, the middle child suffered a lack of oxygen at birth and experienced learning difficulties. When she turned twenty-two, I noticed she was gaining weight. The doctor confirmed my suspicions; she was pregnant. She gave birth to a baby girl and the doctors told us the baby's chances of survival were slim as she developed Neonatal Septicaemia.

The baby recovered enough for us to bring her home and we christened her Amy Jade. Stacey lived at home and I took on the role of caring for Amy. We had two years and nine months with our gorgeous girl before she passed away leaving a huge hole in my heart. Depression washed over me and I can't say my life has improved since that abysmal day. This, along with past traumas, are the triggers that set me on the road to ill health.

The pains I endure are so severe I am unable to walk. Muscle pains are more of a problem. I have tender areas all over my body. When are the doctors going to take my health serious? They have prescribed gabapentin and two types of morphine which FMS patients receive, yet here I am still undiagnosed. I deserve answers.

My health is deteriorating at an alarming rate and it worries my children. Two year ago, they rushed me to hospital with septicaemia. My daughters quick thinking saved my life. She rushed me to the hospital.

My doctor is unsupportive and unsympathetic towards patients diagnosed with FMS. He treats my individual symptoms but does not recognise this disorder as an illness. I live in pyjamas and spend my days upstairs in my bedroom with the curtains drawn. Ruthless migraines are the bane of my life. These are unrelenting and cause not only a pounding headache but nausea and blurred vision. My memory is terrible. I go into a room and forget why. My life is a living hell! I don't venture out as I am unsteady on my feet and have no confidence. I live a hermit lifestyle. How my life has changed.

I am tired of pain, medication, doctors and I am tired of stress. Life is a struggle. People think I am strong. They voice this often, but I am not as strong as they assume. I am in a permanent battle with my body. As each evening closes, I whisper to myself, "Try again tomorrow, Carol". This gives me hope for the new day ahead.

I am still waiting for a diagnosis of FMS.

# Tina T

By the time I was eighteen I had a husband and two children. I loved life until I discovered my husband was a serial cheat.

After leaving the marital home I moved back to my parents with my two boys. it was then I began to experience a few aches and pains, but I brushed them to one side. In time I remarried and had a further three children. I experienced normality until husband number two began drinking and became violent. At the time I had five boys and a home to organise. I felt trapped in a loveless marriage. The violence continued and I became his punch bag. This atmosphere for the children was tough and my nerves were fragile.

While having a rare night out at my niece's pub I met a lovely guy, Martyn. He showed me how my life could be. After meeting him a few more times, I took the five children and returned to my parents a second time to start divorce proceedings. Martyn and I are still together after twenty-six years.

We made a family home with the children then a terrifying trauma struck our family. One of my boys fell in with a local gang of lads (I can't go into much detail as it hit the national media). This gang of thugs came looking for my older son and when they couldn't find him, they kidnapped his younger brother. When he refused to tell them where his older brother was, they bashed him to a pulp. The police rescued my battered boy from the boot of a car. He brought a chilling message home; they were coming for me unless they found his brother. My stress levels hit a new high.

There was a huge police presence and a court case. I lost both of my boys as the police placed them in protection, and moved them to a secret location along with two of my grandchildren. Their new identities were a secret to everyone including myself. It broke me. You read these things in the newspapers or see them on the television, but you never think it will happen to you. I prayed every day for my lost family.

I moved from Bristol to Weymouth and started again. This is where my pain started, and the trauma of the past years triggered FMS. My whole body hurt, not one inch of me was pain free. I then developed a frozen shoulder and pancreatitis. Several months later surgeons removed my gallbladder and my pain became uncontrollable. I visited my GP often complaining of constant pain. He organised tests but all the procedures returned negative. They diagnosed polymyalgia and plied me with steroids. I assumed it was PTSS, but the experts disagreed.

Four years later I received a diagnosis of COPD, but by then I was at a breaking point. I needed answers yet none were forthcoming. Restless legs were and still are the bane of my life along with a host of random symptoms that FMS throws my way. I get dressed if I am going out otherwise, I stay in pyjamas.

Martyn doesn't understand my illness. It's so frustrating but my granddaughter now lives with us. This solution is a huge help. She sorts out my medications and makes sure I take it at the correct time. She also helps around the house with chores.

Floods of tears consume me when my breathing problems and FMS collide. I often shout out, "Why me" but then a voice in my head whispers, "You can do this". I have learned to listen to my body and to the inner voice which encourages me to fight.

It's a pleasure to say I am back in touch with my children and grandchildren, but it's been one hell of a ride and cost me my health. Just telling my story has me in floods of tears. Recalling the past is reliving it all over again. I have been through so much during my life and I am sure if I if I can overcome such trauma, I can fight FMS and its coexisting disorders.

When I am low, I remember this quote. "*We may be broken, but even broken crayons can fill a page with glorious colour*". This encourages me to fight on and live life to the max on a good day even if it means I pay the price later. *Fibro Warriors* deserve colour in an otherwise, "black and white" world.

# Myfanwy

Myfanwy was one of nine children. She often experienced pain as a child. Her insensitive mom thought she was an attention seeker and paid no heed to her complaints. She recalls her mom being a spiteful and heartless parent, so she turned into a withdrawn child who kept things to herself for fear of a scolding.

When Myfanwy turned five. she fell off a wall and fractured her skull. It is her belief this incident along with a callous parent started her lifelong journey of physical pain.

She found her GP apathetic, so she changed to a more understanding doctor. She told him her symptoms which were many and he arranged tests. It was a long-drawn-out procedure of seeing specialists, doctors and trying new medicines.

She knew something was wrong, yet no answers were forthcoming. Myfanwy experiences times when widespread pain engulfs her. When this occurs, she curls up in bed. Other times she talks herself into getting up and attempts to go out. This depends on how she feels each day, as no two days produce the same symptoms. Her medications cause further complications. She takes seventeen tablets a day. She believes the vast volume of medication, including morphine patches cause unwanted side effects and make her existence hell. Memory loss, vertigo, irritability, frustration and sleep deprivation are just a few of the problems she experiences. There are many more to add to her list. She is weary and in agony, but this lady still smiles and gets on with life the best she can.

Myfanwy received a diagnosis of FMS nine years ago. She is now sixty-three years old. It did not surprise me when she admitted she felt everyone, including the NHS failed her. She has lived most of her life in pain.

I have never met this lovely lady; we became friends after talking on an internet page. Despite her disability, she fights to find a path through her pain. Her ability to make everyone laugh astounds me.

She is a true Fibro Warrior.

# Lisa H

My younger years were fraught with anxiety. My mother and I had to flee from an abusive father. We moved into my grandparent's home and I changed schools. This change in the family circumstances caused anxiety. I struggled with depression and became a victim of bullying.

When I turned fifteen. I was taking recreation drugs which began with smoking weed and taking amphetamines. Then I introduced coke and ecstasy to my drug regime. After this, I became dependent on crack cocaine and my life was one big mess.

I turned my life around when I reached the age of twenty-seven, but I still wonder if this twelve-year habit caused emotional or physical damage to my body.

I have been clean now for fourteen years and I am proud of this. Once I was drug free my future looked brighter and I became the primary carer for both my Nana and Grandad until their deaths. The bond we shared was unbreakable, but I couldn't grieve. To keep my mind occupied I threw myself into work as a support worker, but every night I came home and began drinking alcohol to block out the pain.

In October 2018 I called into my neighbour's home and fell down a flight of stairs injuring my back. I went to work as normal the following day but couldn't manage my shift due to severe pain. I was taken to hospital. The doctors informed me it was a severe sprain and gave me Co-Codamol. Two days later I suffered a huge mental breakdown. It was obvious my life events had caught up with me. The bullying, the abuse of my body, the death of my grandparents and widespread pain had rendered me into a total wreck. I couldn't cope with my life. My GP prescribed antidepressants. These helped with low moods, but the pain continued and become more widespread.

Various tests followed and in February 2019 my GP diagnosed me with FMS. It was a relief that my illness had a name, but the relief was short lived. I discovered this was uncurable and a lifelong disorder.

I tried to help myself by quitting cigarettes, I ate healthy and used herbal and natural remedies. I also stopped drinking alcohol.

I take several prescribed medications, some help but it's all trial and error with FMS treatments.

It's ironic I get control of my life and FMS gets a hold of me. I am not telling my story to gain pity or for attention, I am telling it because it's a huge part of my life and I want other people to know you can overcome hurdles through strength and determination. Looking back over the years I realise I lost myself for a long while and that's fine, because I know I came back stronger

# Conclusion

*Everyone, fighting this invisible illness is a Fibro Warrior.*

It would take the hardest of hearts to be unaffected by the traumas our "Fibro Warriors" have endured. What we can take from this is, whatever adversities life thrown our way we can move forward. There is no right way to cope with FMS. We each must find a suitable path through the pain and discomfort as we never know from one day to the next what this disorder has in store.

You are not alone on this journey. There are various groups on Facebook or online which offer valuable information, advice and friendship. I recommend the following groups which have been an asset when I have experienced low mood days. We each are different in how we cope with pain and other comorbidities. Joining online communities and fellowship with other FMS sufferers, is an uplifting experience which is vital to your well-being. After all, who can understand your frustrations better than another sufferer.

FIBROMYALGIA AND CHRONIC ILLNESS FAMILY UK. (Facebook Page)

MOTORBIKERS COSMETIC COMPANY (Facebook Page) This group goes live every week. It's a good support for FMS sufferers. They sell their products worldwide. I have used several of their holistic treatments and found them to be excellent. They are the only distributor of the famous "**Pain Slayer**".

# Further Reading

www.nhs.uk/conditions/fibromyalgia

www.health.com

www.healthline.com

www.fightfibromyalgia.net

www.fmcpaware.org

https://fibromyalgiaresources.com/the-7-stages-of-fibromyalgia

www.webmd>fibromyalgia

www.everydayhealth.com/fibromyalgia/does-your-family-get-it

www.everydayhealth.com/fibromyalgia/myths-facts-about-fibromyalgia

www.nrshealthcare.co.uk/articles/condition/fibromyalgia

www.webmd.com/fibromyalgia/guide/fibromyalgia-in-children-and-teens

Printed in Great Britain
by Amazon